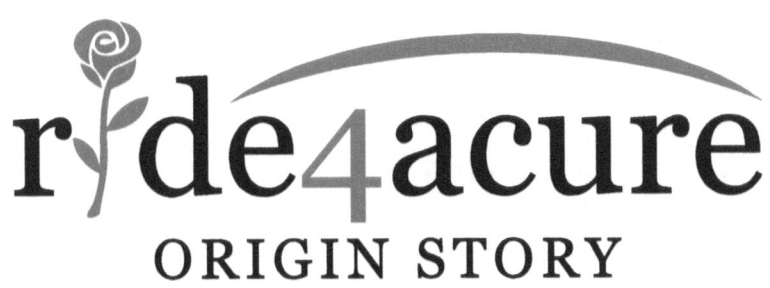

ORIGIN STORY

...hope, love, resilience and grit...

MAURA LUXFORD

First published by Ultimate World Publishing 2024
Copyright © 2024 Maura Luxford

ISBN

Paperback: 978-1-923123-88-5
Ebook: 978-1-923123-89-2

Maura Luxford has asserted her rights under the Copyright, Designs and Patents Act 1988 to be identified as the author of this work. The information in this book is based on the author's experiences and opinions. The publisher specifically disclaims responsibility for any adverse consequences which may result from use of the information contained herein. Permission to use information has been sought by the author. Any breaches will be rectified in further editions of the book.

All rights reserved. No part of this publication may be reproduced, stored in or introduced into a retrieval system, or transmitted in any form, or by any means (electronic, mechanical, photocopying, recording or otherwise) without the prior written permission of the author. Any person who does any unauthorised act in relation to this publication may be liable to criminal prosecution and civil claims for damages. Enquiries should be made through the publisher.

Cover design: Ultimate World Publishing
Layout and typesetting: Ultimate World Publishing
Editor: Vanessa McKay
Cover Image Copyright: Back cover image Photographer is Casey Micallef Photography - https://www.caseymicallefphotography.com.au

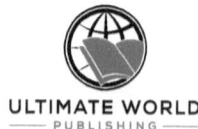

Ultimate World Publishing
Diamond Creek,
Victoria Australia 3089
www.writeabook.com.au

Testimonials

Maura Luxford is one of the bold brave hearts of our time. This book is a rural family story, embedded in land and life. Maura's writing is rich with evocation, storytelling that takes us to places none of us want to be, and places everyone wants to be. Maura is a born storyteller. I felt the earth beneath my feet, the sunshine on my face; smelled the campfires and listened to the soft nicker of horses. Readers will find it a privilege to live this deeply human journey.

Dr Stephanie Dale
International Wellbeing-through-writing Institute

Above all, this is a compelling love story. About the undying love between mother and daughter, between family and community, for country and this temporary earthly life and something more enduring that lies beyond.

Maura lays herself bare during the most excruciating time of her life, and in doing so we get to bear witness to her mettle and tenderness as she transforms pain into purpose.

ride4acure ORIGIN STORY

The book offers us all the gift of transparency. When we share and show of ourselves in our darkest times like Maura has, intimacy between one and many is forged. I now feel I know this woman and her world, intimately.

I didn't want to put the book down, nor did I want it to end.

Thea O'Connor
Wellbeing & Productivity Advisor, TEDx speaker, Coach
Founder of Menopause at Work® Asia Pacific
Creator of NapNow - normalising the powernap as the new coffee break.

Maura Luxford is the embodiment of love. The way in which she has navigated her daughter's untimely passing turning tragedy to powerful action is an inspiration to us all.

Over the many years I've known Maura she's always been the first to give to others even when she's had very little left in her own tank. A kind, thoughtful and incredibly empowering woman, this story carry's lessons we can all learn from.

Maura has a magical way of turning negativity to positivity and that's exactly what you'll get on reading this important book. Maura puts life's challenges into context and provides some important tools to live a whole and rewarding life.

Kerry Grace
CEO Evolve Network

Testimonials

Maura Luxford's first book "ride4acure-Origin Story" is a heart-filled account of her family's journey through the life and death of her first-born and forever-loved daughter Hannah.

Maura shares exquisite details of the life that she and her family enjoyed and endured, allowing us to imagine how we might respond if faced with the news of a sudden devastating cancer diagnosis.

Maura's love for animals, county life and community shine through and create mental images that allow us, the reader, to feel the love and grounding that Maura has. This makes it possible to gently absorb the universal reminder…that we have one life and we are not in control.

"So much unknown. I felt like I was in a game of whack-a-mole… What this story of love, loss, grief and hope boils down to for me is the moments in life where we choose what action to take."

I feel grateful to know Hannah through Maura's words, and I am forever grateful that Maura penned this account. I commend it to you, with the knowledge that in reading it, you will experience the love and universal human connection that is life … and loss.

Jessie Williams
Manager Community Care Programs Northern Beaches

ride4acure ORIGIN STORY

Oprah Winfrey said, "Whether you flounder, or flourish is always in your hands – you are the single biggest influence in your life. Your journey begins with a choice to get up, step out, and live fully." Maura is such a woman. When her eldest daughter died, I witnessed her unquestionable authenticity. She lived the rawness of grief, with robust honesty. Over thirty plus years, I have never seen her lose her capacity to be the protagonist of her life. She takes what comes and turns it into an opportunity for learning and possibility. From her generous heart she takes the lessons of life and uses them to enhance the lives of others. As a mother, psychotherapist, community woman, horsewoman, educator, innovator, and gardener, she shows seemingly endless energy for seeing potential and converting it into building what is good in the people around her. To me she is inspirational.

Father Chris
Chaplin MSC

It takes an immense generosity of spirit and unshakeable integrity to share something as intimate as the life, the death, and subsequent grief for your beloved daughter. Maura's story is not bleak. It is joyous, full of love and deeply affirming. It's about connection. It's about seizing the moment. it's about listening deeply to the world and saying 'Yes'. I love this book. It's brave, important and compelling. Just like life should be.

Mandy Nolan Comedian
Writer and Activist

Dedication

*To all hearts who know the searing ache of loss,
may you find a seed of peace within these pages.
For my beloved daughter Hannah Rose till we meet again.*

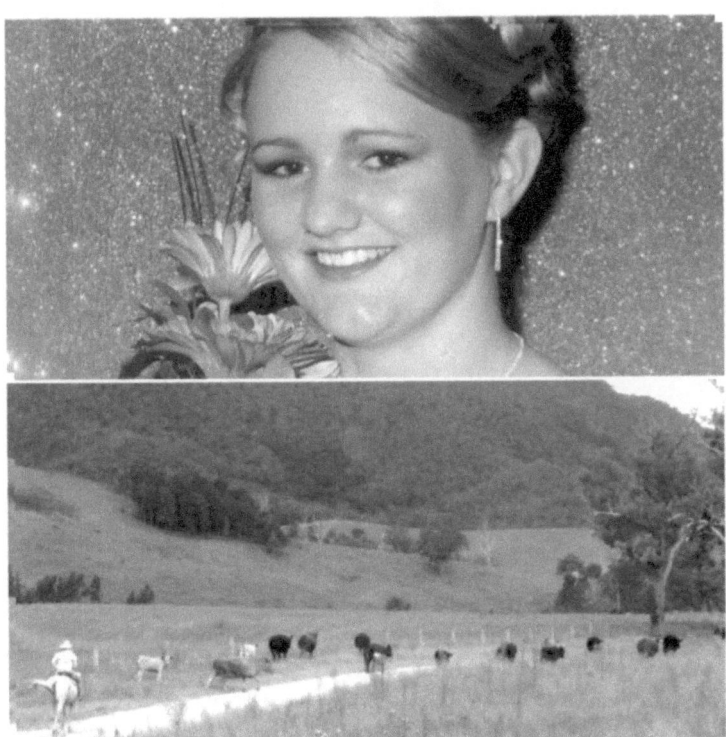

Top: Hannah's 2006 St Paul's Deb photo
Bottom: Hannah on Lena mustering
on the farm at Tait's Creek

Contents

Testimonials	iii
Dedication	vii
Foreword	1
Introduction	5
Chapter 1: Hat Trick in Life	7
Chapter 2: Fresh Start	17
Chapter 3: Just Watch It	21
Chapter 4: It's Back	37
Chapter 5: Doctor Google - Not Just a Cyst	45
Chapter 6: When we get Through This Thing	51
Chapter 7: My Radiation Dog	55
Chapter 8: Groundhog Day	59
Chapter 9: Making the Most of Every Moment	69
Chapter 10: Focus on What's Under Our Noses	75
Chapter 11: Burnt to a Crisp and Free	79

ride4acure ORIGIN STORY

Chapter 12: Another Universe	87
Chapter 13: Trying for Normal	91
Chapter 14: Eulogy Flow	131
Chapter 15: The Wake	145
Chapter 16: Gap Month - Ellenborough River	157
Chapter 17: Returning Home	161
Chapter 18: A Man is Not a Financial Plan	169
Chapter 19: Beyond Grief	177
Chapter 20: Talking About Our Dead	181
Chapter 21: Lighthouse Moment	185
Afterword	199
Acknowledgements	203
About The Author	209
Book 2 Due Out Summer 2024	211
Speaker Bio	213
Book Club - Questions for Readers	215

Foreword

Maura's story is a powerful example of the enduring strength of connection, the fragility of life and the power of love. A natural storyteller and teacher, Maura writes about the origin of ride4acure, formed after her daughter Hannah died at just 20. My initial encounter with Maura's remarkable work and the mission of ride4acure dates back to 2012 at the Sydney School for Social Entrepreneurs. I was a student in 2010, starting a health promotion charity, creating new conversations about loss and death. It made sense that we would have similar interests, and Maura, by this stage, was re-developing the education materials for Mela-What? and working to redefine her role in the Hannah Rose Melanoma Research Fund. In meeting Maura, I learnt that she had already provided education to over 20,000 students and young people, not to mention her presentations to health professionals and community groups. I deeply admired Maura's passion; she was a magnet for partnerships. Maura got things done.

ride4acure ORIGIN STORY

In the pages that follow, Maura invites us into the experiences that inspired ride4acure. This includes the people, places, landscapes, and animals that shaped this astonishing story. Above all, Maura describes how, as a family, Hannah, Esther and Joe navigate the doctors, treatments, and hospitals to make a meaningful life. Holding on to normality, the things that matter, and the things you can control, like taking one step in front of another. There are no cliches in this story, as Maura has a tender way of bringing us along on this journey. And there are many paths! OR should I say the many rides! The car, truck, bike, and horse rides. In all this movement, there are lessons about the nature of grief. Yes, it's a kick in the guts. Yes, it immobilises and takes us to the ground. Yes, it is undeniably a whole-body experience. And it is also a lived experience – an "alive" experience, so even when our hearts are hurting, somehow our bodies move.

We need human connection, love, and kindness from our community. Maura's story also demonstrates the importance of compassionate healthcare and a supportive workplace. For health professionals, it is a reminder that patient and family-centred care must be our priority because when we get it right, and are led by patients and families, it profoundly impacts on how people die. There really are no do-overs when the people we care for need a timely diagnosis, or indeed if they are in the last few days of life.

For families who have or who are currently facing serious illness together, this book will be deeply relatable. There is comfort in a book that can so adequately describe how

Foreword

life, amidst the complexity of serious illness, somehow continues. Maura has a knack for focusing on the things she can control, simple things like connecting with nature or watching DVDs on repeat. Or deciding when Dr Google is no longer helpful.

While I was reading, the word 'grit' kept coming to mind. An unwavering in the face of exhaustion and sorrow. There are joys and challenges, and yet Maura conveys a sense of hope that it is possible to keep moving onward, step by step, into life without the people we love. I encourage readers to let this book be a reminder that grief is not something to be feared or avoided, but rather part of the human experience.

Dr Kerrie Noonan
Clinical psychologist and social researcher
BA(Psych) MPsych (Clinical) PhD
Death Literacy Institute

Introduction

Stealing my sister's brand new book as a four-year-old then hiding under a bush to lose myself in the pictures, became my first experience of inspiration.

Seeing and feeling that hint of a future for myself, outside the present moment.

Nearly sixty years later that inspiration has never left me. At times it may have felt a little distant, however I found my way back home to it. My path home has and is always through being connected and grounded in nature.

Writing the origin story of ride4acure has been like sitting at the kitchen table with you, my readers. I've wanted to deliver on my promise to share the bones of this story. The origin of the ride4acure story is rich with simple moments of inspiration told through a mosaic of memories. They are memories that have risen from the ashes of my own grief journey.

This story of love, loss, grief, hope and grit boils down to moments in life where I had to choose what action to take. That action has changed the course of my life and the lives of others.

Looking back now, I'm grateful that when I was at the t-intersections after loss, I said "Yes". Hundreds of people have shared their stories of loss and grief with me, often buried deep for decades. I know firsthand how healing it is to have someone simply be alongside me, even a stranger, and listen.

What has unfolded for me happened one step at a time, one choice at a time.

The grief journey is personal, unique and there is no road map. One description that I've leant into is the image of our fingerprint. It's ours alone. Not comparable to others. Grief can look similar to someone else's journey but in essence is our unique blueprint.

The most authentic statement said to me during the fresh years after Hannah's death were people who simply said, "I don't know what you're going through, but I'm here."

Chapter 1

Hat Trick in Life

Double-barrelled numbers are powerful.

The year I turned 44 didn't disappoint.

Winter 2006 was my hat-trick of life-changing events. Within twelve short weeks, I navigated a total hip replacement. Mum's death. My marriage ending.

It was the closing chapter on what had been a rich time of my life.

Our home was Mount Sebastopol, Moparrabah, west of Kempsey, nestled in the foothills of the Great Dividing

ride4acure ORIGIN STORY

Range, a magnificent place of cultural significance. Majestic limestone escarpments, unique caves and incredible rainforest, with an ancient white fig tree in the heart estimated to be hundreds of years old.

It is wild mountain country, with its towering limestone escarpment and dramatic cliff face. Our farm was a parcel of land of over twelve hundred acres. At the foot of the cliff face sat two hundred acres of rainforest with the pristine waters of Tait's Creek running through the centre. The area was abundant with animals and plants.

The farm was just under fifty kilometres from Kempsey, half of that was rough, dirt-corrugated road. The farm was the backdrop to our lives for over a decade. A paradise and playground for the kids, David and me.

When the kids and I weren't at a horse event somewhere, the weekends would include a ride to the rainforest and the Bullock Paddock. It was a wild ride with some treacherous trails for the horses. Steep ridges that took us to the boundary fences. Once off the creek flats, we'd follow narrow tracks that were formed by cattle bashing through the bush and lantana to reach spring gullies of fresh feed.

As often as we could, we'd ride our horses to the rainforest, a couple of kilometres from the saddle shed, criss-crossing the creek, riding through gullies and bands of rainforest hugging the creek banks. The creek banks were a riot of lilli pilli trees, brush box, mountain ash, coachwood and some corkwood forming a thick protective barrier to the rainforest. It was full of ferns, fig trees, elk and stag horns perched on rocks, with a towering ancient fig in the centre standing as a guardian of the forest.

Abundant wildlife was everywhere. Goannas skuttling up trees as we rode by, wallabies, the occasional dingo and snake sightings along creek crossings. We loved it when the lilli pillies were fruiting as we'd ride alongside and feast from our saddles.

We would tie our horses to the fence posts at the gateway to the rainforest, as it was impossible to ride safely through it. Massive vines were twisted into ropes and strung between trees. Some huge vines, as thick as human arms, hung invitingly for people to sit and swing on. Scattered throughout were the infamous stinging trees. The stinging hair from this tree would be painful for days or even months, with the hairs penetrating deep into the skin of humans. The kids were taught early never, ever touch a leaf. We told the kids the sting is worse than a thousand stinging nettles. Our kids didn't, but their friends sometimes did. Luckily a big sappy plant with leaves shaped like droopy elephant ears, unsurprisingly called elephant's ear, grew in the creek and was an antidote to the sting.

The paddocks on the farm were fertile creek flats, covered in a variety of native pastures, peppered with spring gullies that fed underground waterways. The strong green stripes across the paddocks showed our eyes when the water table was up as the grass was brighter, greener than everywhere else. There were limestone rocks scattered throughout the farm. The kids gave some of the rocks names. Including one of our favourites Pride Rock. This came about one day when we rode through the Orange Tree Paddock, our smallest dog Michelle a Jack Russell-Chihuahua-Fox Terrier cross, ran onto this rock protruding a metre out over the water in Tait's Creek. She lifted her little front foot while looking poignantly into the distance. We were stock still watching her and the other dogs. The kids said she looked like Mustafa in the Lion King looking out over his kingdom. Michelle was surveying her queendom and from that day on we called it Pride Rock. Rocks featured on the farm with massive conglomerate rocks dotted throughout. It was a walk-through time with fossilised remnants to remind us that this was all once the ocean floor.

There is a challenging ride above Spring Gully that would take us up the mountain where majestic rock overhangs were. Smooth areas of closely cropped green mats of soft carpet grass were at the foot of many limestone walls of rock. It was easy to imagine a time before settlement, when women and children would have gathered there to rest.

These places connected us to life before colonisation. A few hundred years ago, when Dunghutti tribes called this place home and were custodians of the land. Standing or sitting anywhere on the farm put me and many others in that mindset. It was impossible not to feel connected to Country and feel the life once lived by First Nations people.

Hat Trick in Life

Our farm was the classroom for my work for TAFE NSW where I delivered dozens of programs using horses. Many Dunghutti Elders worked with me as mentors, and community members came to the farm. This was a significant thing and played a key role in the farm being sold to National Parks to expand the Willi Willi National Park, which is now protected into the future as part of the World Heritage site Gondwana Rainforest of Australia.

When not working or at school, we were riding horses. We always had horses handy to ride anywhere on the farm, or to neighbours who lived kilometres away. We used horses for all our farm jobs. Mustering, checking cattle, or just for fun, we'd pack saddle bags with matches, newspaper, bread, frozen sausages, tomato sauce and sausage wires. The kids made the sausage wires from plain fencing wire, with a twisted handle to get a good handhold. The simple process of sliding a sausage on the wire and cooking over the fire was so satisfying. Joe was doing this from two years old; it was his favourite way to eat.

In the first few years of living at the farm, the twice daily trip to the McKenzie's Creek school bus stop was nine kilometres of narrow, winding corrugated dirt road from the farm each way. The bus left at 7.30am for the journey into Kempsey to school. It was the longest bus route in the Macleay Valley and the roughest. I think our bus driver had a special spot in his heart for the McKenzie Creek kids. Once a term, our bus driver would organise with the families to arrive half an hour early and light a campfire and cook sausages for brekky.

ride4acure ORIGIN STORY

The paddocks were all named. Road Paddock had a public road called Willi Willi Road running through it for about a kilometre. When we first moved to the farm in 1997, a busy traffic day was two cars coming through. David had been living on the farm for twenty years and there was a big heavy, wooden gate at the boundary. Cars had to stop and open and close the gate. I've never been a big fan of opening gates and when David asked me to marry him and we moved up to the farm, one of the first things I put into action was getting the gate converted to a cattle grid at both boundary fences on Willi Willi Road.

Other paddock names on the farm were The Mountain Paddock, Spring Gully, The House Paddock, The Horse Paddock, Orange Tree Paddock and the Bullock Paddock. The Horse Paddock had the cattle yards which were a hundred years old and made from locally harvested tallowwood timber. They had stood the test of time. I extended them to include horse arenas, and a saddle shed, which was the outdoor classroom for my riding school I established called Full Circle Horsemanship. I taught horsemanship courses for Kempsey TAFE for seven years in the early 2000s.

I worked from our farm and had built a series of arenas and my office - The Saddle Shed. It became my home away from home. I loved to be there as I felt deeply connected to country and it evoked a sense of profound peace. I had a deep passion for my work and experienced a sense of flow. I delivered a constant stream of programs during holiday periods, privately with community service organisations, school groups from regional areas and groups from Sydney in partnership with the Redfern Community Centre for young Aboriginal learners.

Scattered across the farm were over a hundred mapped limestone caves. David was a keen speleologist and was an active member of the Kempsey Speleological Society that is Kempsey Caving Club. The club would regularly meet at the farm and explore the caves and map new ones.

Several universities came and undertook research into interesting fields like grass trees, native snails and rare plant species. They would camp up at the Horse Paddock and many times from about the age of five, Joe would want to camp with them. He was always practicing setting up his own tent in the backyard and then around that five-year-old mark got brave and asked to set his tent up when the grass tree uni people were there for a few days. The lead researcher had her eight-year-old daughter with her and Joe asked if he could set his tent up near theirs. It was over 250 metres from the house. He bravely took his camping gear to the yards and set his tent up; he then spent the first of many nights there. At his birthday parties over the years, he would camp with mates down there and with the caving club.

The Saddle Shed area was beside the arenas and stockyards. There was a pit dunny (toilet) about fifteen metres away from the shed discretely nestled in behind rocks and a few trees. A lean-to off the side doubled as our classroom and meeting room. It had a long redgum table with stools that could seat a dozen people. Alongside the shed were a variety of large rocks that students sat on. There were big logs set up on limestone rocks as seating. The saddle shed was made of corrugated iron, and housed a huge amount of saddlery and equipment including over twenty saddles and all my teaching equipment. Near the table was a camp fire area to cook and boil the billy. It was the ideal 'primitive' camping place and classroom. Over three hundred students came to the farm to study natural horsemanship over seven years.

The Farm for many years was paradise for my kids and me. Until it wasn't.

In the middle of 2006, I had a hip replacement that saw me in hospital in Sydney for two weeks, then in rehabilitation in Kempsey for a few more weeks. This was a massive disruption to our lives as a full-time working Mum with three kids at school, involved in several businesses, my own business, Full Circle Horsemanship, teaching for TAFE, and doing the bookwork for our joint business Collett Vegetation Management; it was a hectic time.

All this while Hannah, my first-born daughter, was in her final year of high school. My eldest sister Yoni had generously come to support my family for the time I was in hospital. David, my husband, had a business doing contract vegetation control that, during its peak, had up to eight full time employees.

The three months following surgery were life changing for me and my family. A month later, Mum died and a month after that, a decade after moving to the farm, it was untenable to stay. The three kids and I left in mid-September and moved to a small 25-acre property at Temagog near the Macleay River, 20 kilometres from the Tait's Creek Farm and for Joe, still on the same bus route.

Joe told his teachers and school friends we'd moved to town. That was because we now lived on a bitumen road and had a garbage service! We were still twenty-five kilometres from Kempsey.

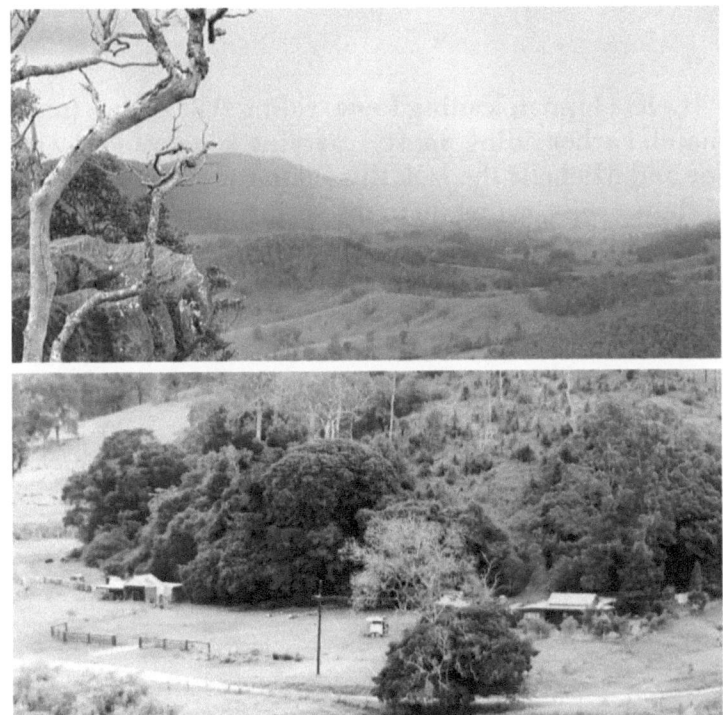

Top: View from Mount Sebastapol
Bottom: The farm, Taits Creek, Moparrabah.

ride4acure ORIGIN STORY

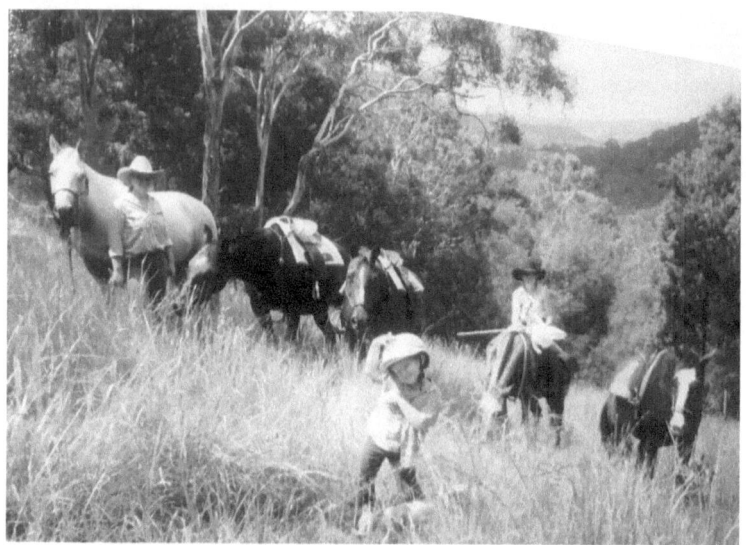

(L-R) Hannah leading Lena, riding Ally; Rosie (my mare), Esther riding Spotty, carrying Clancy (dog) with Joe and Michelle the Jack Russell in the foreground and his horse Billy, riding up to the spring gully on our farm.

Chapter 2

Fresh Start

By springtime we had settled into our new home. A two-storey rustic red cedar house nestled amongst a eucalypt forest of grey gums and tallowwood trees. A small creek flowed through the heart of the 25-acre property.

Hannah was finishing high school and planning to attend university the following year. Esther was in Year 10 and Joe in primary school.

I had landed in nirvana. Each morning I would walk the boundary with the dogs, greeting birds and wallabies. They would scamper out of my way into the undergrowth, seeking invisibility. The horses would be in formation plodding behind me in single file, meandering along the track through the bush until they found a patch of sweet green grass that quickly refocused their attention. When the horses stopped to chew grass, I would pause in that early morning light, close my eyes and listen. The dogs would come close and sit at my feet and I would focus all my attention on the sounds I could hear. I loved the sound of the horses tearing the sweet, soft grass with their teeth and grinding it in their mouths. The feeling of all that horse and dog energy around me was sublime. It buoyed my spirit in ways that sustained me. It was a dose of medicine that strengthened me to navigate my life. It was a time to gather my thoughts for the day before the sun was up, pre-dawn, a drover's favourite time. As I walked, I breathed the promise deep inside of what opportunities lay ahead for me and my family. I was in my happy place with all three of my kids home.

Full-time work with TAFE NSW consisted of coordinating and teaching horsemanship programs for youth at risk and teaching in humanities, community services and disability discipline areas. As a newly single mother of three kids, business woman of Full Circle Horsemanship, buying and selling horses and supporter of my kid's horsemanship goals, my life was rich and full. Both the girls bought and sold horses too and there were always deals being done. Most weekends, the kids and I would load the truck or horse float up and head to horse events. They were family time for us. We loved camping and being around other families with the same passion. Esther was an A-grade showjumper and eventer and both girls were keen competitors in

Fresh Start

campdrafting. All three kids competed in pony club and mounted games. For two years before Hannah died, Esther was Zone 9 Pony Club A-grade eventing champion, and Hannah was the Under 21 Zone 9 Campdraft Champion.

Each year in winter holidays, the kids and I would pack up and head off on the Junior Rodeo Circuit. It was the highlight of our year and a time where we made deep shared happy memories together. Some years, my nieces and nephews came and joined us. It was a week or so of travelling, camping and competing across the Mid North Coast. We started with St Paul's Rodeo in Kempsey, Nabiac, Wingham, Bulahdelah and Gloucester Junior Rodeos. It was always freezing, with plenty of frosts, with savage ones at Gloucester and Wingham.

Joe loved setting up camps from the time he could walk. All three kids loved the planning, packing and the logistics of camping. It was never a chore to help. They loved it as much as I did. From around the age of three, Joe took on the responsibility of *guardian of the campfire*. He'd collect dry sticks and firewood for the campfire weeks before we went and stack them into a chaff bags. At the time, it didn't feel like a lot. It simply felt like our unique life. It was rich, fulfilling and rewarding. Life was rich and we felt free and happy, living at Temagog.

ride4acure ORIGIN STORY

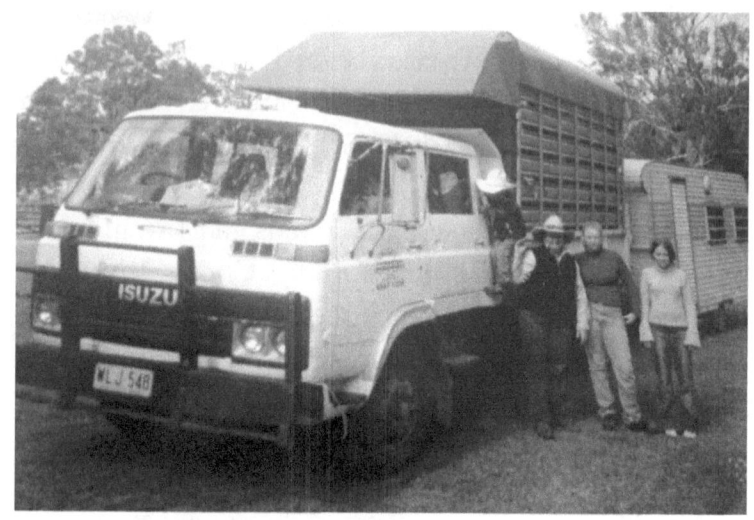

Junior Rodeo time, loaded and ready for the road.

Chapter 3

Just Watch It

Hannah's university experience was peppered with fake sick medical visits, not because she was sick but purely to get medical certificates for assignment extensions to submit after the due date. This was because she was off at a campdraft or rodeo and needed extra time to submit her papers, not because of her health.

The two times that mattered to me I found out after the fact in November 2007. Unbeknown to me, Hannah had six months apart, asked two doctors about a spot that had appeared under her ear on her neck. Both said to watch it. Early November 2007, Hannah was home from uni for a long weekend. We'd been out mustering cattle all day.

ride4acure ORIGIN STORY

When the livestock and horses had been taken care of, we'd gone back to clean up and cook dinner. After our showers, I was giving her a shoulder massage and facial, and while massaging her neck felt the slight roughness of a spot and for the first time saw this new mole like an 'orange spot' and asked her about it.

"Hey, this spot is new. I've never noticed this before," I said.

"Yeah, it came up six months ago, but don't worry Mum, it's nothing. I've asked two doctors and they both said to watch it," Hannah said.

"Has it been itchy?" I asked.

I was feeling it and looking at this friendly little spot, but something deep in my gut was telling me it wasn't ok. It felt rough on top and a little dry to my touch.

I felt a strong pull in my gut that it wasn't okay. I was feeling roughness to my touch and could see it was several colours of orange. I didn't know much about skin cancer but I knew itchy, rough and new were signs to get a spot looked at.

"Well, I don't like the look of it and I'm booking you into Carmel for a skin check in a fortnight when you're next home." She was heading back to the University of New England in Armidale, a three-hour drive from home the next day.

Just Watch It

A fortnight later when Hannah was home again, I was preparing my Diploma of Community Services students for their graduation and end-of-year celebration. Hannah, Joe and I had driven to town together, and we dropped Joe at his school. We pulled up at TAFE and she came in and said g'day to the staff in our shared office. My kids spent a lot of time hanging out at TAFE waiting for me to finish work to get a ride home rather than catch the bus. Joe had a side-hustle selling his fresh eggs to staff. He would write messages on the cartons in his spidery handwriting. *Eggs from Joe's Happy Hens.* It seemed to me his little scrawled messages were a value add for the buyers.

This day I was a matter of fact about how the day would go. Hannah would take herself to Dr Carmel Shanahan at the Kempsey Skin Cancer Clinic for a routine check. I'd had suspect spots removed and send to pathology to check their status. I had no reason to think Hannah's visit would be more than that.

Two hours later a distressed Hannah was standing in my office doorway. There were several other staff in the shared office. Hannah had a large dressing on her neck under her ear and she looked directly at me, and a girl who hardly swore said,

"They cut half my fucking neck off!" And burst into tears.

I went to her and hugged her. I took time off work to run her home to Temagog. It was a twenty-minute drive each way. I got Hannah settled with snacks, set up on the couch for an afternoon of TV watching, and went back into work at TAFE for the rest of the day.

Joe and I arrived home late afternoon to find Hannah asleep on the couch, with Australia's Next Top Model softly playing on the television in the background. A large white fluffy Persian cat was fast asleep on her chest purring away. Only thing was we didn't own a cat; we had a crew of dogs that had never seen cats. Perhaps a problem. This was a total left-field surprise. Joe and I were standing bug-eyed near Hannah, staring at her and the cat. Joe giving me side eyes, trying to work out what had happened. Neither of us dared to move in case we woke her or the white fluffy cat. Joe was as shocked as I at the size of the dressing on Hannah's neck.

Our laser-like staring finally stirred her, and she slowly opened her eyes. A slow, smile filled her lovely face, causing us to spontaneously smile back at her. It's hard to express how much we loved Hannah. She was such a deeply gentle soul, with a depth of kindness and love that we all craved more of, with every cell of our beings.

Hannah had a way of gentling things down. To say she loved all creatures is an understatement. When she was two years old and her dad Lindsay and I were droving in Western NSW, she collected a colony of hairy caterpillars that she kept in a small box with twigs and dry grass. There was a dozen of them and every day in the caravan she would meticulously line them up on the kitchen table and sing to them for about ten minutes, then carefully put them back in the box and go about her day. They all had names, and she was adamant they were all different. When she was little, she often would stand stock still, and when I'd get close to her, I'd see a butterfly had landed on her and she didn't want to scare it. This fascination with nature and animals never left her.

Joe and I were standing, absorbing the picture of her and the fluffy white cat.

Hannah didn't move a muscle as she didn't want to disturb the cat.

"When you dropped me home, mum I went to the bathroom, this cat was curled up on the dryer, waiting for me. I think God sent her," Hannah said.

We didn't argue with that.

The cat stayed. The dogs didn't go near it in the house. Outside, it was fair game. Inside, it spent all its time purring on Hannah's chest.

The next morning at 7am, our phone rang. It was a busy time of the day. I'd already been up for two hours. Outside jobs done. Morning ritual walk around the property for half an hour, done. We were all getting ready and Hannah was going to relax at home again. I had a graduation and last day of the Diploma course with a group of fourteen dedicated students. Esther was away working for Olympic eventing coaches; Joe was getting himself ready for school and feeding animals though he'd tried to scam time to stay home with Hannah.

The call was from Dr Carmel Shanahan. I asked questions about the size of the biopsy and questioned her about taking such a big sample.

"Maura stop talking and listen, I mean it," Dr Carmel said emphatically. I did.

"Maura, whatever you've got on today, cancel it. You need to have Hannah and yourself in my clinic by 8.30am. Not negotiable. See you then," she said matter-of-factly. No room to answer her, as she had hung up on her last word. She was as pragmatic as me.

I slammed the wall phone back in its hanger and had a rant to the kids about fucking doctors over reacting.

I was saying to myself, *I can't change my day. It's not that easy. I've got an end-of-year graduation.* Deep down I was rocked. Something wasn't right. What doctor demanded a mother and her daughter to her clinic like that? What for? It couldn't be that bad. She must be overreacting. I had to hide my concern from the kids. So I did.

"It's okay you lot. Carmel's probably overreacting. We'll do what she says, but it's probably nothing," I said with as much conviction as I could muster.

Just Watch It

Hannah's relaxing day on the couch was thrown out the window.

Dressed and in the car with us again, we headed off to the doctors in Kempsey. A repeat of the day before.

I had to go to TAFE to let my head teacher know what was going on.

"I need to sort the doctor out and I will be back at TAFE mid-morning and we could have the graduation then," I said to her. How naïve I was.

Hannah was calm about it all. I asked her how she was feeling and she said, "Okay, not too worried, like you I think she's overreacting."

When we arrived at the clinic, Carmel's administration person, waved us straight through to the consulting room. The look of concern and empathy she gave me put me on edge, increasing the creeping feeling that something was out of whack.

"I'm going to cut straight to it Hannah and Maura," Carmel said directly to us both, then her eyes went to Hannah and stayed there.

"Hannah, there's no way to say this easily. You have a very serious melanoma. Stage 4. I have made arrangements for you in Sydney tomorrow to see a leading melanoma surgeon who will perform surgery to remove the affected area. You will need to stay in Sydney for a while," Carmel said.

Carmel looked me straight in the eye for a nanosecond then gave Hannah her full attention.

"How can I have melanoma? Only old people get that," Hannah said.

I was dumbfounded. I literally couldn't speak. My words wouldn't come. My brain was like mist in my head. I couldn't find my thoughts. It felt like a sliding doors moment. I'd stepped into someone else's life. What were Carmel and Hannah saying? I couldn't hear them. I had this foghorn going off in my brain that was draining their words out.

Silence filled the room. I could hear the murmurings in the distance. A huge heavy silence filled my brain. No words made it to my mouth.

What felt like an hour was only a few minutes.

I came back to my senses and realised the room was silent. Both Dr Carmel and Hannah were looking at me, waiting for me to respond.

I knew I had to get myself together. Get present.

"Okay Carmel, what do we need to do to get through this?" I said and reached over and held Hannah's hand.

Just Watch It

Carmel stepped us through the plan and what we needed to do. She had made all the arrangements. Her calm, coordinated and confident manner gave us hope.

Carmel clearly explained that surgery was the first step. The surgeon was a leader in melanoma and she assured us Hannah was in a safe set of hands. This surgery was to remove the melanoma and get clear margins around the site to ensure the cancer hadn't spread to her lymph system.

Round one in Sydney was a blur. I had to organise kids, livestock, dogs to be fed, time off work, leaving the house for an indefinite amount of time. I didn't know when I'd be back in Kempsey. Fortunately, as a family from the bush, I had good friends in Sydney, Adrian and Jeannie, that we could stay with. Adrian was the priest at Christ Church Saint Laurence in George Street Sydney. Jeannie had been Esther's home-birth midwife back in 1990 and we'd remained friends for life. Staying with Jeannie and Adrian felt like family and softened the edges of the whole medical journey for us. Jeannie lovingly prepared meals and always had beds for us.

Christ Church Saint Laurence is a heritage-listed building in the heart of Hay Market Sydney. A three-story timber and brick building built to survive and to emanate a sense of grandeur.

Sweeping stairways, high vaulted ceilings, massive rooms. It was a million miles from the home among the bush back at Temagog but it was a haven for us. A shelter from the chaos and noise of the city and a peaceful reprieve from the turmoil of a health crisis.

That Christmas was to be our first Camp Luxford. We'd been planning this family event for a year, however, with Hannah still in Sydney waiting for outcomes from surgery, we didn't know if we'd get there or if she'd need further treatment.

The idea of Camp Luxford came about after Mum's funeral when my eight siblings and I were talking on the footpath at the front of our sister, Kate's home in West Melbourne; we talked about bringing the family together. It's what Mum had done consistently and so well throughout all our lives. We felt compelled to do this and began planning for the first Camp Luxford. Here we were over a year later, wanting with all our hearts to meet up with all the clan at Eagle Point, Victoria, for five days over Christmas. My kids and I had been excited all year. They loved mixing it up with their cousins, and this was a whole-scale Luxford Clan experience.

Three days before the Camp Luxford kick-off, we were waiting in Sydney, post-surgery for the all clear for Hannah to leave. I did a ten-hour, round-trip drive back to our home at Temagog, in the spirit of the best outcome. Before results were known. I energetically wouldn't accept 'any other outcome than all clear'. I'd been saying to Hannah all along, you will be okay. You've got this. We've got this. Mentally, none of us would entertain any other outcome

Just Watch It

than 100% healing. When I arrived home at Temagog, I packed all our Christmas things. Our Holden Jackaroo was loaded to the hilt with presents and all our gear. Nine-year-old Joe and seventeen-year-old Esther decorated the bullbar of the 4WD with tinsel and reindeer antlers and we set sail back to Sydney to our Hannah with Six White Boomers and the whole mix of Aussie Christmas Carols blaring in the CD player. I acted as if it all was going to be okay and the kids took their lead from me. I simply didn't let an alternate future exist. That was my truth.

Mindset matters to me. It matters in every element of my life and never more than when I was walking with Hannah through her year living with melanoma. Two thoughts that were on loud speaker in my brain that year were that our *thoughts become our words and our words become our actions* and *our energy follows our focus*. A horseman told me a brilliant story that stayed with me not only training horses and dogs, but also aligned with my kid-raising ethos and guidance for tough times. The story goes there was a horseman riding and came across a Native American cowboy carving wooden Indians and he had them for sale. There was a row of identical six-inch-high carvings lined up. The old horseman had stopped his horse and marvelled at how they were all exactly the same and asked the carver, "How to you make them 100% identical?"

The carver replied, "I simply carve away what doesn't look like a wooden Indian."

ride4acure ORIGIN STORY

Hannah, Esther, Joe and I believed wholeheartedly that Hannah would be okay and that we would go to Victoria for our first Camp Luxford with all our family. Our job was to carve away anything that didn't look like being with Hannah, together with her big crew of cousins and family at Camp Luxford.

It was a ten-hour driving day for me to go home and return to Sydney, plus the Christmas packing in the middle. I was running on pure adrenaline. Par for the course the whole year.

The surgery was complete. We were waiting for the results of the margins to return without a trace of melanoma. The surgery and treatments are tough, but the waiting is edgy. It was a constant challenge to remain in the moment and focus only on what we actually know. It felt like a million times a day I was telling myself to "not shoot until I see the whites of their eyes". This was a saying my dad, Kevin Luxford often said to not put energy into the unknown. This was the tough part of not being in our own environment.

At home there are distractions. Horses, dogs, gardens, cooking. In Sydney it was trickier, so we watched the dozens of dodgy DVDs we'd bought from the highly illegal DVD shop above a travel agent near Central Station, which had a handwritten cardboard sign taped to another sign that said, 'DVDs' and had an arrow pointing up stairs. This trove of media delights came at only $2 each for the latest release movies. Given we were on the tightest of budgets, this was a bonus for me.

Just Watch It

The room where the DVDs were sold had a dozen copying machines set up in full view of customers. Only one person had a bit of English to deal with the money side of things. Hannah bought chick flick movies by the dozen. We watched every single one of them over and over. Hannah and I curled up on the double bed with snacks and drinks, and a dozen pillows and cushions watching until our eyeballs hurt and we'd doze off. Hours passed somehow.

After the quick dash back home when I got back to Hannah in Sydney, we still had 48 hours to wait for the results. The kids all piled into the bed and watched DVDs. Esther and Hannah now sending Joe downstairs for snacks and drink refills. It was incredible to be back together. We were a tight unit, the four of us. We were all different yet perfect in our family huddle.

Finally, the day came - 22nd December 2007 - for the appointment with the surgeon for the results. If it was all clear, we could go. If the margins showed signs of melanoma, we would have to stay for further surgery, radiation and consults with a medical oncologist.

Here we were on that day, standing in the surgeons' clinic and he put a hand on each of her shoulders and said, "Hannah, you're the luckiest girl alive. You're all clear. Go home and tell all your friends to look after their skin. Hannah and I both burst into tears and hugged each other." The relief was palpable.

ride4acure ORIGIN STORY

When we got back to Adrian and Jeannie's, they were all gathered in the small dining room off the kitchen and Hannah shared her incredible news. Within an hour, we were on the road to Victoria and our first Camp Luxford.

Driving away from Sydney, we slammed the door on that chapter of our lives. We truly felt blessed, lucky, that we could get back to normal. That Christmas we celebrated life, being alive, having a future surrounded by a big, wild family. To go from a month of being in Sydney, marinating in a medical and surgical soup to the freedom of a holiday at Camp Luxford with all the clan was incredible and burned into our hearts and minds forever. We didn't know how precious the memories would be.

Looking back, I realise we all took it for granted that this would be the first of many more Christmases with our Hannah. Oblivious that one year later on Christmas Eve, we would be at her funeral.

The Camp Luxford site at Eagle Point was well set out a couple of hundred metres from Lake Victoria. It was originally used as a school camping site. It had a large commercial kitchen and dining room. Games rooms and units for each family group to stay in and a couple of large dormitory rooms that older cousins could cram into. Best of all, an outdoor fire pit to gather around. There were about forty of us that first year. Food preparation was massive. Full Christmas menu and loads of it. Kate (our family chef) managed the kitchen and we took turns and supported her.

Just Watch It

Part of the dining hall was set up with several game tables for cards, board games and a jigsaw table. There was a constant game of cards on the go and even as adults, plenty of argy-bargy about rules.

We were loud, feisty, sometimes argumentative, but we were family. We were together as a family for the first time since Mum's death. She had instilled in us the value of showing up. After the last month in Sydney, it was the perfect remedy and reminded us all of what was most important.

Chapter 4

It's Back

After Christmas, life quickly returned to normal. Hannah went back to uni in February and decided to study by distance and get work in agriculture in the Riverina. She continued to do well with her course work and life went on. In our minds we had thought melanoma was a one off. Hannah was throwing herself into life. Barrel racing and campdrafting on Lena as often as possible. Time with friends and family. Life was good. She had her own Commodore ute and horse float and was independent to travel to events.

Hannah was passionate about barrel racing and, most weekends was heading off with her cousin Bec to a competition. One weekend, she was having a run at Digger's

ride4acure ORIGIN STORY

Rest at a Turn and Burn event. I was 1300 kms away when late on Sunday afternoon I got a phone call from Bec.

"Aunty Mauz, sit down," she said.

"What's going on Bec, tell me." I demanded. I knew in my gut something was wrong.

"Hans had a bit of an accident," she said. "We were at Diggers Rest rodeo and at the end of her run coming home, her girth gave way and she collected a fence post and broke a few bones."

"She is in an ambulance on her way to the spinal unit in Melbourne now," she said.

Within half an hour of receiving the phone call, I was on my way to Newcastle Airport, a four-hour drive from home to get on a standby flight down there. That was the quickest option for me in the bush. Hannah had eleven fractures to her vertebrae, a broken leg, shoulder and collarbone. A 'bit of an accident' was an understatement of the year.

When I finally got to Melbourne and walked into her room, she was lying flat out, high as a kite on pain medication and beaming from ear to ear. She was so happy to see me, and almost the first thing she shared with me was how good her run was, how well Lena went up till it wasn't and the girth gave way. She didn't remember much of the crash.

It's Back

One of Hannah's nurses was completing her masters with a research topic of reoccurrence of cancer post trauma. I thought it was interesting and when she told me, I felt a chill in my spine.

When Hannah was through the worst of it, she could be discharged, but only to a home that could take a wheelchair and had a bathroom toilet that could have a shower-toilet chair. That ruled out family in Melbourne. One of Hannah's rodeo friends had a farm that was a couple of hours from the hospital. She was happy as a bug to be there with them, and she was in great hands. I left a few days later as it was clear she was going to be ok and was on track for full recovery. Aunty Veronica was keeping an eye on her. It was good for her to be around horses and people that had a passion for the things she loved. It helped accelerate her recovery.

A couple of months later, I received a phone call from Hannah at the end of July 2008.

"Guess where I am Mum?" she asked.

I could hear the sound of a vehicle engine and a lot of road noise.

"No idea, surprise me," I said with a droll tone in my voice as I suspected I would not be thrilled with her response.

"I'm in a truck loaded with horses heading to Mount Isa Rodeo!" she excitedly responded.

ride4acure ORIGIN STORY

I was silent. Pin drop silent in my head, processing in tiny detail how her recently fractured and still recovering body was taking it easy and how had she stretched and pulled herself to get herself up into a truck, and the impact on her recently broken bones and bruised muscles. There was no way any truck going from Victoria to Isa was stopping every couple of hours for her to stretch and relax her beautiful body. Long driving hours cramped up as a passenger. It was one of many defining moments where I accepted, she was a young adult making choices for herself and I responded in the only way I could that gave her autonomy.

"I trust you to make wise decisions, Hannah."

I felt a deep silence, endless silence inside my mind. It was a defining moment. I had let my eldest daughter lead her own life. She was studying at uni, working and travelling on her own terms. I had to give her the space to make choices, live her life, and love her whether or not I agreed.

That she'd had two life-threatening moments in six short months gave her every right to do, in my books, the outrageous. She was right to not tell me until she was committed to a trip in a truck carrying horses, driving 24 plus hours to a rodeo on roads through outback Australia. The nurturer, safety keeper in me, was tense and held back a lot of my thoughts about the choices she was making. My problem, not hers. I listened to words about, "An opportunity too good to miss"… "Aunty Veronica is gonna keep an eye

It's Back

on me" and "I will be camping with her…" I had a million questions, but they weren't hers to answer.

Hannah was to be in Isa for the rodeo for a couple of weeks and was excited and happy. A few days into being there she told me she'd met a cowboy called Darcy and they got on really well. Hannah had been checking out the broncs and bulls while wandering around the rodeo. She was watching a young cowboy feed the bulls. He approached her and they clicked. From the moment they met, they spent all their time together. Yarning endlessly for hours on end. Watching the rodeo, feeding bulls, playing cards and generally hanging out together. I was happy she had a guardian that was watching out for her. She was loving the rodeo, and it inspired her for her own future as a cowgirl dreaming of the day she'd ride there herself.

August 6, Esther's eighteenth birthday, I got a phone call. I thought Hannah was calling to talk about Esthers' eighteenth birthday. I was sitting in my office at Kempsey TAFE.

"The lump's back Mum, right in the same place as the surgery. I don't think it's anything, but I wanted to tell you. It is the size of a plum," Hannah said.

Her voice had a slight stretched quality to it, her pitch higher than usual. I could feel her unexpressed anxiety down the phone, though when I asked her how she felt, she dismissed it, saying it was probably a cyst.

ride4acure ORIGIN STORY

I did a quick Google search looking for a doctor in Mt Isa while listening to Hannah talk about what was going on. She sounded light-hearted and not too worried. My fingers were going lightning speed. There was half a dozen, and I simply landed my finger on one and wrote the number down.

"I've found a doctor and I'm going to hang up from you and make an appointment and I will call you back in a few minutes."

I quickly called the Mount Isa Doctor. I asked the receptionist if I could speak to him directly as I had an urgent request. When I explained the situation, she made it happen. Unbelievably within a few minutes I was speaking to the GP. I explained to him Hannah's two high-risk health experiences in the last six months and that I wanted him to assess her and while he's doing that, I would set up a teleconference with both Dr Carmel Shanahan in Kempsey her diagnosing GP, and her Sydney melanoma specialist. The kind Mt Isa GP asked me for more information about Dr Carmel and it turns out they went to university together. It felt like a sign things were okay.

Somehow all that came together and before long we were having a five-way conversation. Me in my TAFE office in Kempsey, Hannah and the GP in Mount Isa, Dr Carmel Shanahan in Kempsey and the melanoma specialist in Sydney.

It's Back

All I remember from that conversation was her specialist saying to Hannah, "Hannah, you need to come to Sydney for me to examine you as soon as possible."

"I've waited my whole life to come to Isa; it's probably only a cyst. And I don't want to miss this," Hannah responded.

"If it's a cyst Hannah, I will personally fly you back to Mount Isa!" he promised.

The disappointment in Hannah's voice was palpable from two thousand kilometres away.

Thank God for the internet because by the time the teleconference was ending, I had Hannah's flight from Mount Isa to Sydney booked and texted through details. There were only two flights per week. The next flight was two days away. I was arranging my work to leave to get to Sydney to be there with her.

"Make the most of the next two days, Han. Everyone is working together to make sure you're going to be OK," I said.

"I'm deeply grateful to everyone on this call for coming together to help Hannah and us, her family," I said, without bursting into sobs.

I waited till I hung up the phone and cried my heart out at my desk. My line manager, was there. She gently put her hand on my shoulder as I stood up and I collapsed into her with a hug. I cried more. I couldn't fathom what had just unfolded and that potentially the melanoma was back. I was gutted. The wind was knocked out of me for a moment. I cried until my tears dried up. And then a wave of gratitude washed through me, as I was so grateful for the incredible people who were helping us navigate this horrendous road through what was happening in Hannah's body.

Again, I heard Dad's voice say to me, *Mauz, don't shoot till you see the whites of their eyes.* Get a hold of my mind. Stay focused only on what I know. What I knew was that there was an incredible group of medical people who cared about getting the best assessment and, if needed, follow-up treatment for my daughter.

I had a stone-cold feeling in the pit of my gut telling me it was not a cyst. Hannah's next two days were filled with the rodeo, watching her Aunty Veronica and her cousins ride and connecting deeply with her love of this sport. She loved the dust, heat, wildness of it all and the people. Rodeo people are a special breed. People who live for their horses and livestock, travelling huge distances to compete. It was all part of the experience. And of course, she was on the cusp of a romance with Darcy, and in Hannah's words, he was *one hot cowboy*. I was thinking he turned up at the right time and was good medicine for her.

Chapter 5

Doctor Google - Not Just a Cyst

This potential reoccurrence was a shock to me. It showed me the line in the sand. I had believed with all my being that the melanoma had been a one off. I thought the process was diagnose, cut it out, clear margins, then that's it. After all, 'she was the luckiest girl alive', we thought. This proved otherwise.

Two major medical incidents in six months and here I was, lining up for a third. So much unknown. I felt like I was in a game of whack-a-mole. Life-changing moments could pop up and knock us down with no warning. In an instant we had to pivot, adapt, make plans and take action. It evoked in me an axis-shifting wariness about the unexpected. Life hit me with surprises. A bizarre game with strong odds against us. A game with complex and deadly consequences.

I contrasted this melanoma journey to our ordinary family life, my work and community life back in Kempsey.

I was thinking in my darkest times, *why us, why my daughter?* There was no room for those thoughts to take up space in my mind or heart. When they arose, I quickly processed them through journalling or realigning my mindset and energy. I was relentless at weeding out thoughts that didn't serve my own mental health and my kids. I didn't dwell on what we had no control over. We were in unfamiliar territory and had to trust an ever-increasing team of health professionals to light the way through this dark night of the soul. Hannah and those of us closest to her, had full faith she would recover and continue to live a bright, full life and have the life experiences she had her heart set on.

In the year Hannah lived with the recurring melanoma and the fracture fiasco from Diggers Rest, she never once complained, blamed or lost faith that she would be okay. She never said to any of us, "Why me?" She held onto the life she loved with a fierceness and kept focused on the fantastic future she planned for herself. Her belief, like ours, was strong. Hannah was as fully alive as a human could be while living with a life-threatening disease.

To not slide into an abyss of despondency, I had to keep my mind focused on one thing at a time. What's the next step? Who is involved? What do I need to put in place to have a successful outcome for Hannah? Do it. One step at a time. I wasn't thinking long term. *What is under my nose today?* was my most common thought. What requires my focused attention now? Do it and move on. Repeat that process again and again and again.

I called Jeannie and Adrian and explained what was on the cards and they generously opened their doors to us again. The next day, after yet another a five-and-a-half-hour drive from Temagog to Sydney in my Ford ute, I landed at Jeannie and Adrian's to prepare for Hannah's arrival and *round two* of what was next.

"Jeannie, can I use your computer?" I asked.

Yoni, my eldest sister, was an academic at the University of New England in Armidale and was in Sydney for a conference and staying with Adrian and Jeannie too. Yoni and Jeannie are both nurses with stellar careers in their respective fields. I didn't dare tell them what I was going to do.

"Sure Mauz, go for it," Jeannie said.

I traipsed up to the third floor of the presbytery to Jeannie's study. The sound of their animated happy voices sharing their news followed me up the stairs. When two midwives are in the same room there is always a lot to talk about.

ride4acure ORIGIN STORY

Climbing the stairs there was dark toned wood everywhere, with magenta carpet cascading down them. The church and presbytery date back to 1845. The timber was logged over two hundred years ago in Tasmania and featured throughout the home. Staying in the presbytery was a step back in time, an immersion in history.

Sitting in front of Jeannie's computer, I Googled, "Stage 4 melanoma in young adults."

I was breathless as the hundreds of hits filled the screen. Cold as ice, I was shocked by the details and dismal prognosis laid out before me. I felt hopeless at that moment. The life knocked out of me. Gut-punched. I cried my heart out sitting on my own in that third storey study. Dr Google was serving me up endless pages of doom.

With the wind knocked out of me, I felt hopeless, defeated; that melanoma was too insidious. This thing that can grow unknown and wreak havoc in a young, healthy woman without warning.

Hannah didn't use any of the common language associated with a cancer diagnosis. She didn't fight, battle, war against cancer. But in that moment for me it felt like my enemy. This insidious cellular growth trying to establish itself in my girl's cells.

Hannah focused on life, energy, love, healthy cells. She had a laser like-vision marinating in positive energy, seeing, feeling and believing that the cancer cells were decreasing, diminishing, disappearing. She was led by the outcome she wanted, not amplifying what she didn't want. This helped her stay happy, grounded, alive, and engaged while navigating a cancer experience. She would often say to people when they referred to her as being sick, "I'm not sick. I just have cancer."

I thought of all this, of the path Hannah was carving for herself and that I was called to stand with her, as I sat in a midwife's study. A room with amazing posters and artwork on the walls celebrating women's bodies, midwifery and birth. Here I was doomsday dwelling on the worst-case scenario of my precious first born daughter's life. I made a steely decision in that moment that Dr Google wasn't my friend. That was the one and only time I searched for a prognosis.

I quickly shut the computer down and made my mind up; that would not be Hannah's story. She was going to be the exception. I decided I didn't want to know everyone else's story and that I'd be guided by Hannah's needs at this time. Hannah was 100% focused on her recovery and the daily steps she needed to do that. My role was to support her wholeheartedly. I would ask the medical team better questions and be guided by Hannah.

I walked slowly and heavily down the three flights of stairs to the kitchen where Jeannie and Yoni were making tea. They took one look at me and knew what I'd been up to.

Jeannie was graceful in her response to me. Affirming the will in me to know more, but the risks of taking on information that was out of context for Hannah's experience and mine as her carer. It was what I needed to hear. She mentioned talking with her if I wanted help and we could look together at reputable research and outcomes. I valued this guidance as the internet was a rabbit hole and I didn't have the energy to waste if it wasn't going to support where we were at.

Each time I left home at Temagog to support Hannah, Joe lived with his dad, David, up on the farm at Moparrabah. Esther was away working for Olympic eventing coaches. She periodically came to Sydney to visit us when she could in her little 'Beep Beep Barina' car. A small Holden vehicle that was super economical. It cost the equivalent of a motorbike to run. Perfect for Esther, who lived on a tight budget. Each time Esther visited, Hannah asked endless questions about all the horses she was working and how her own horses, Diva and Titan, were going. Hannah was invested in Esther's eventing career and dreamed with Esther of one day riding for Australia.

Chapter 6

When we get Through this Thing.

As horsewomen, we'd had a level of fitness that supported our work with horses and livestock. Strong women, who could lift, pull, reach, balance. We felt physically strong, capable, resilient in all situations. However, in the twelve months Hannah navigated having melanoma, both our fitness levels wavered until by the end of that first year I'd gained twenty kilograms, lost a lot of my strength. Months of long bouts of waiting in hospitals and clinics. Knowing that Hannah was yet again having another lifesaving intervention. For a year, I barely slept. Hannah and I had exercised together for years as an aside to horse-riding, including jogging and swimming.

ride4acure ORIGIN STORY

Many times, throughout her stays in hospital and particularly her last, she said to me earnestly, "Mum, when we get through this thing, let's get fit again."

"I promise we will, Hannah my darling, but let's focus on getting you well again, eh," I said lovingly.

Hannah was in and out of hospital four times in that year. Both in Sydney and Melbourne. As a second year Bachelor of Livestock Science student at the University of New England, she was juggling a full-time course load and practicals. I was a TAFE NSW Teacher and Course Coordinator, Director of Full Circle Horsemanship and single mother to three kids.

The blessing buried deep in this tumultuous year was sitting in the fire of life and burning the dross away from what was life sustaining and what wasn't. I learnt that year to pick things up, invest as much as was possible, and put them down again. I became a ninja at this and my team at TAFE were incredible. All my colleagues knew and cared for my kids, as they'd spent so much time at the campus in Kempsey after school.

I learnt through blood, sweat and many tears to let go of what I couldn't influence and control. My number one focus that year was to be present to Hannah and nurture and support her to the best of my capacity. And I did.

When we get Through this Thing.

Besides the mainstream medical support, Hannah actively consulted with naturopaths and acupuncturists. These modalities helped enormously with managing side effects and optimising her own innate capacity to heal.

I was blessed with my work teaching for TAFE. My line manager and institute director were all supportive and understood the unpredictability of my life and were flexible and supportive. I felt a load of guilt that I wasn't there to nurture my students through their courses. I loved teaching. It was in my blood. I was passionate about my work and loved the interaction with students and respected being a part of supporting life-changing educational opportunities for people.

Hannah was looking forward to two major horse events that were on Esther's radar. Zone 9 One Day Event Championships at Nana Glen near Coffs Harbour and the NSW Pony Club One Day Event Championships at Wagga Wagga.

Hannah was staunch that she would get to both no matter what. It gave her so much joy to watch Esther and Diva compete. Esther and Hannah shared such a deep love and passion for their horses and sport.

Chapter 7

My Radiation Dog

Hannah and Esther would talk for hours endlessly about how Diva's training was going and her up-and-coming eventer, Titan. Hannah was invested in every detail. Esther was in training for the Zone 9 NSW Pony Club One Day Event Championships at Nana Glen and this was her second year of competing in A Grade. She was hoping for a repeat and a win.

Her next goal after that was to get to the NSW One Day Event Championships that were to be held in Wagga Wagga a month after Nana Glen. That would be the biggest event Esther and Diva had qualified for. Esther had got her red p's licence, which enabled her to tow her own horse float, which was a bonus during this time as I would be back in Sydney with Hannah for the months of radiation. Esther needed my ute to get herself and Diva to Wagga. We had a Kara Kar angled two-horse float that was brilliant to tow. It would be Esthers' first long trip and she would tow her own horse through Sydney. I had a lot of faith in her capability as an eighteen-year-old. Luckily, my three kids were all at the motor registry, as close to their birthdays to get their licenses. Like most farm kids, they were driving vehicles as soon as they could reach the steering wheel and clutch pedal.

After returning from Mount Isa Rodeo and the second round of surgery, Hannah had to wait for the surgical wounds to heal and undergo significant physiotherapy before the commencement of radiation.

The planets aligned for us as Zone 9 NSW Pony Club One Day Eventing Championships at Nana Glen were scheduled during that time. My eldest sister Yoni came to Sydney and picked us up and took us to Nana Glen. It was around a seven-hour road trip each way.

On arriving at Nana Glen, Esther had an area at her camp set up with a swag so that Hannah could have naps whenever she needed. The previous month in Sydney had been exhausting.

We were sitting at the camp and I noticed a woman walking around with a large cane carry basket with a lid

My Radiation Dog

that folded back into the middle. Out of one end of the basket were half a dozen tiny little furry Jack Russell puppy heads.

I saw the woman walking through the crowd and went to her and asked if she could bring the puppy basket over to show Hannah. We were a Jack Russell family and this basket of puppies were adorable. As we walked together to where Hannah was resting, I mentioned what Hannah was going through at the moment and what was ahead. She was only too happy to bring the puppies to her.

The woman sat the basket next to Hannah on the swag and Han woke up. When she saw the pups, she reached out for one in particular to pat his little head, asking if she could hold it. The woman said yes and Hannah picked this little pup up and gave it a cuddle. Within a minute, the pup is curled up on her neck right where her scar was and hung its legs on either side of her neck. Hannah was smiling from ear to ear, laying there and said, "Look, it's my little radiation dog."

The kind woman left the pup there with Hannah for hours on end and it never moved, just laid there until it was time to walk the course with Esther. Hannah insisted on doing that even though she didn't have that much energy. She mustered enough to walk slowly around the course, still carrying the little pup.

Hannah kept asking me if she could buy the puppy. The woman had already told me that all the pups were sold as they were pedigree show dogs. I asked the woman for her contact details and tucked them away in my phone.

There was excitement that day as Esther did well in all three events, dressage, showjumping and a clear round in the cross country. Esther and Diva were magnificent and won the A Grade event, making it two years in a row. Hannah, Joe, and I were so proud of Esther and Diva for their efforts. We were excited then about the NSW Championships at Wagga in a month's time and Hannah was already saying to Esther that no matter what, she would be at Wagga to watch her.

Chapter 8

Groundhog Day

I met Hannah's Mount Isa flight at Sydney airport. I was standing at the bottom of the escalators as she came down. She was lit up with light, energy, and happiness, wearing her hat and boots. Her rodeo gear bag was dumped near her boots on the escalator step. As I watched her descend to me, I thought, *how could something sinister be potentially growing inside my daughter?* It was a mercurial story unfolding. She looked amazing. We hugged for a long while.

Then I said in a hurry, "Airport parking. We need to rock'n'roll out of here, Hannah."

Airport parking was ridiculously expensive. Every cent mattered to me. I was juggling a monetary tight rope with expenses.

Another quote Dad used to say to me often when I first started working for him at fourteen was, *Mauz, look after the pennies and the pounds look after themselves.*

"Let's get out of here, Han," I said and off we went back to Jeannie and Adrian's.

I didn't comment on the sight of the plum sized lump on her scarred neck. But there it was. Huge, imposing. Impossible to miss. Hannah had a cotton scarf wrapped around it, but I could see it when I was up close.

Tomorrow we would begin the journey again, back on the merry-go-round of medical appointments, tests, and waiting. We would soon know the current state and steps to healing. That was our focus.

"Can we find time to visit the Dodgy DVD shop and stock up again, Mum?" Hannah was quick to say.

When she said this, I knew she knew in her gut it wasn't a cyst. She had mentally prepared herself for what lay ahead again.

"We will make time, Han," I said and reached out and took her hand as we walked back to the ute.

Groundhog Day

Within 48 hours, Hannah was in hospital again for more complex surgery. The rapid growth of the tumour was not good news. Hannah had said it had come up almost overnight. This time the melanoma had spread into her lymph nodes in her neck, armpit and chest.

The doctor explained that some major nerves would be lost in the surgery required to remove the lump and the nodes. It would result in loss of some function in her left arm and shoulder.

"So long as I can lift my arm to chest height that's ok. I need to be able to saddle my own horse." Her priorities were set right there.

Our optimism had taken a kick, however I kept digging deeper every moment. I simply wouldn't allow any thought other than complete healing to occupy my mind. I was resolute. Hannah was in the same swim lane. She saw herself fully recovered. Healthy and happy.

My mind returned to the nurse at the spinal unit in Melbourne who was doing her masters on the reoccurrence of cancer following trauma. Could it be related? I made contact with her and let her know that Hannah's melanoma was back so soon after the fractures.

The surgery was gruelling. This time, Hannah had to stay in the hospital for a week. She was in a shared women's ward. At twenty, she was the youngest by twenty plus years. Several of the women were in their eighties and in a lot of pain. The room reverberated with the sounds of women in pain.

In the bed next to Hannah was a mum, early forties, with three teenage sons who faithfully visited her daily. It was a joy for Hannah to see the boys. She chatted with them as they were around her age. Esther had come up from the Hunter Valley. Yoni and Jeannie were daily visitors. I never left Hannah's side.

On day three, the mother in the bed next to Hannah died while her boys were visiting. Right there in the room. The boys were distraught, and so were we. I realised that regardless of the medical reasons for being in the hospital, the emotional roller coaster of being in a ward with extremely ill people was a game changer.

Hannah asked me repeatedly, "Could that happen to me Mum?"

It was impossible to overcome the emotional load that was in that ward. I immediately made an appointment to see the social worker. I wanted to explore getting Hannah moved elsewhere, away from end-of-life risk. The constant sounds of pain from the older women and this death were game changers for us. Our mental health was at risk.

It felt like we were marinating in death soup being in that ward. The mum had been awake and animated and when her kids weren't there, she talked with us. The other older

Groundhog Day

women seemed in pain all the time and never slept. They were groaning frequently, and the sound penetrated into both our minds and hearts. I was feeling for these women and all those confined to hospitals. So detached from ordinary life. This ward was no place for an otherwise healthy twenty-year-old girl to be. Hannah had noise cancelling headphones on to drown out the hospital sounds. But I knew in my gut and heart this was no place for healing.

Hannah had to remain in the hospital for infection control. She had what we lovingly called her handbag. A large drainage bag hooked up, draining fluids from her chest that went everywhere with her. Yoni, Jeannie, Hannah and I met with the doctors and the social worker. We proposed that, as Yoni and Jeannie were both professional nurses with a lifetime of experience, to get permission from the team for Hannah to be nursed at home at Jeannie and Adrian's rather than stay in hospital. It was close by, only a suburb away if there was an emergency. Permission was given. This caused great joy between us and felt like a win. How naïve we were!

The surgery was only step one. After the wounds healed, she was scheduled for a month of daily radiation. But our focus couldn't go there yet, we had to keep focused on what was in front of us one day at a time, an hour at a time, this minute. This helped Hannah and I, and both Joe and Esther, stay focused.

Ten-year-old Joe gave Hannah regular reports of how boring school was and his antics riding his motorbike on the farm and the caving adventures he had with his dad David, and the Kempsey Caving Club.

Joe had a gift of sharing stories that made Hannah laugh. He noticed the little things about people, the environment, and animals. He had fun making up stories about his life to share with Hannah. It broke my heart as he asked every time when we'd come home. He came to Sydney a few times to visit Hannah flying from Port Macquarie to Sydney. It was tough for him to see this version of his Big Sis. This version of Hannah was radically different to him from his ordinary one. She ruled his world and had a love for him that was unique. She was tough with him too. If Joe did things that didn't align with her version of an awesome little brother, she would stand in her tough-love place and pull him into line. Seeing the Hannah we knew and loved, having to keep showing up for treatment and radiation and watching her decline, was tough on us all. Hannah was adamant she was going to be ok. There was no space for maudlin thinking and she banished all thoughts of not getting well. Our mantra of the wooden Indian guided our mindset every minute of every day for those months.

Our lives shrank over the next few months. Life at the presbytery was rounds of sleeping, eating and a blur of phone conversations with medical people, family and friends. The daily grind of radiation was an alien way of living. Life during this time felt like we had been kidnapped and taken to a secret location and dropped in a strange environment.

Groundhog Day

Medical events prior to melanoma were the odd trip to fracture clinics. We were a family that didn't get sick. Hannah loved correcting people; she wasn't sick, she just had cancer. She loved her body and took a lot of pride in her nutrition, movement and how she looked. She loved to have a vibe with her clothes because it made her happy. Loved a quirky hat and scarf. Sydney living gave her an opportunity to give that a workout. Every day, even though she had such a finite amount of energy and her body hurt beyond words from the radiation burns and constant fatigue, she took time to dress in a way that made her smile.

I wore out a lot of boot leather looking for skin creams that would ease the pain of the radiation burns. Naturopaths made lotions that helped a little bit but the reality was radiation was an assault on her body. However, it was one that Hannah had judged to be worth it, as it was the best option to eliminate any residual malignant cells lurking in her tissues. We tried to reframe the burns as a good sign that the radiation was killing off the cells. The reality was it burnt through her chest to her back and burnt her skin badly. This took months to heal after the last round was complete.

One thing Hannah looked forward to, and would not be told it couldn't happen, was going to Wagga Wagga halfway through the radiation cycles to watch Esther for a long weekend when there was no radiation scheduled. This was tricky as she was exhausted and every effort tired her out. Darcy had followed Hannah back to NSW a few weeks after Mount Isa and got a job on a property near Wagga Wagga. He could get time off work and come and visit while we were there.

We had her swag rolled out in the back of my ute all the time and she napped a lot. She was propped up so she could see out into the camp. Darcy spent most of his time laying with her and they talked endlessly about the life they would build together when this chapter ended. When Esther wasn't riding or prepping, she was laying on the other side of Hannah. Hannah was very much in love with Darcy and often called him her *Sexy Hot Cowboy*. They were always touching, hugging, holding hands. He was the best medicine on the planet for Hannah. He helped her feel her future.

At the NSW Pony Club Eventing State Championship, Esther and Diva represented Zone 9 and had three rounds to compete in. Dressage, Show jumping and Cross Country. In our camp, there was Lindsay, me, Esther, Hannah, and Darcy. When Esther was competing, we all set up to watch and Hannah was on her chair, perched in a prime viewing position. This was one of the greatest joys for Hannah.

Hannah had insisted on walking the course with Esther, Darcy, Lindsay, and I. We took a chair so she could rest when needed. We took the time it took to walk slowly around the course while Esther at each jump consulted with Hannah on how she'd pace Diva for particularly tricky approaches.

Groundhog Day

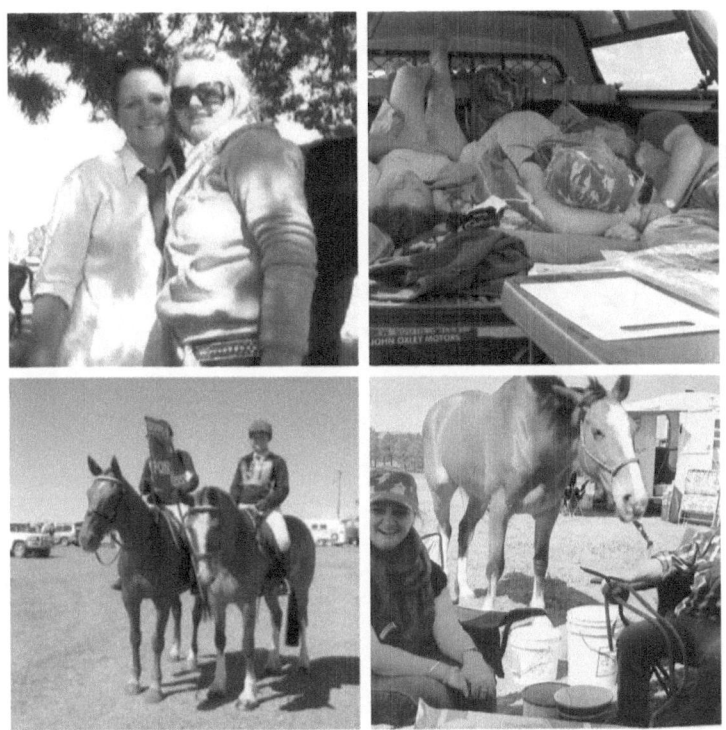

**Wagga Wagga NSW Pony Club
Championship One Day Event
Clockwise from top left: Esther and Hannah;
Esther, Hannah and Darcy; Esther and Diva
(horse on right); Hannah, Diva and Lindsay.**

We were thrilled and delighted when Esther and Diva were in the winner's circle and sashed with sixth place in the top ten riders in the state.

The memories made at Wagga Wagga were revisited often during the next few months. Hannah would randomly start talking about Esther and Diva and how well they went. Esther's eventing achievements gave Hannah a lot of joy.

Hannah had stopped showjumping at C Grade and put her energy into campdrafting and rodeo. Esther relished the challenge of getting to A Grade and the complexity of the higher grades. We were her cheer squad and would go anywhere to watch and support the Esther-Diva team.

Chapter 9

Making the Most of Every Moment

Radiation was the second most challenging period. It was physically horrific. Because of the positioning it meant Hannah's jaw, neck, shoulder and upper chest copped it. She was roasted. The radiation burnt right through her body to her back. The pain of her skin peeling and blistering was hideous. It peeled off like overcooked lasagna sheets.

Hannah focused on healing and getting back to the life she loved. In between the treatments, she was studying and working to fund her passion for barrel racing and campdrafting, rode her beloved mare Lena, and travelled as much as she could.

While frazzled to her core, fatigued beyond comprehension, Hannah wrote lists. She wrote out her schedule for study, how she would catch up. She wrote out what rodeos she'd get to once she was back on her feet. She wrote out a schedule for getting both Lena, and herself fit again. These passions kept Hannah going.

The thing that shocked me most about intensive hospital stays and treatments was the scale of it. Every day there are thousands of Hannahs quietly going about with earth-shattering health experiences that disrupt their own and their family's lives. This had barely made a ripple in my world prior to Hannah's diagnosis.

Her energy was like a beacon. She inspired me to focus on life in the moment. Her persistent, authentic, positivity in the face of life-threatening disorder was compelling. She was my teacher. Her mindset was phenomenal. Hannah focused on what she could influence and let the rest go. The general narrative about having cancer is it's a battle, a war, a fight, a scourge. She saw it as a cellular process with her scientific mind and would kindly tell people, "I'm not sick. I just have cancer."

I learnt in those many moments of being by her side through the tough conversations and procedures that happiness is a decision made in the moment and from within. To be happy while navigating this pathway was some of the defining and great spiritual moments of my life. True self-love. Hannah never gave up on herself. Never blamed herself or spun her wheels in the *'Why me?'* space. Not one single time. Hannah chose life every moment.

I was the opposite. Now and again, when I'd had a gut full of the continuing shocks of that year, I'd rail against the heavens. I had moments of rage at this entity *melanoma*, that had turned my family upside down. I reckon that was healthy. I punched a pillow or two in the privacy of my room to transfer the relentless tightness I felt in my shoulders. A few well directed haymakers into the pillow were better than any massage at releasing muscle tension.

The grind of living away from home was relentless. Leaving paid work for indefinite periods of time and struggling to financially survive, juggling sick leave and Centrelink. On the outside, I was methodical in my mindset. To others, I was coping amazingly well. I was relentless to focus only on what I could influence and not give any air time to 'what ifs' and anything outside my immediate control. However, there were moments when I did a practice I called, 'letting the dog off the chain.' Working dogs go nuts when they're let off their chain until called to, *come behind*. They let off pent-up energy. My thoughts were like that. I'd give myself some private time to let them rip. No filtering or editing. Stream of consciousness pouring out onto the pages into one of the hundreds of journals I kept. Old exercise books, bits of paper, journals I did then and still do, write on anything.

I'd write till my hand cramped and I was exhausted. Then I could rest and recalibrate and reconnect to my priority of keeping love flowing to my other kids, Esther and Joe, who were equally whammed with the road-train crash that is a serious cancer diagnosis. It's an uprooting of family; we felt exposed and vulnerable.

We had to adjust to manage the trips to Sydney and long stays with our good friends, Adrian and Jeannie. Multiple venues to receive treatment. Attend a clinic with the melanoma specialist in one place, radiation in North Sydney. Surgery at Newtown. All of this entailed transport in an unfamiliar city. The months of radiation was a 500-metre walk to Central Railway Station from Haymarket then catching a train to North Sydney. Hannah insisted on walking, even though it would exhaust her. It was her fitness challenge. She would often fall asleep on the train. Then there was a walk up and down a steep hill into the hospital for radiation. We simply took it all one step at a time. We never thought about the destination, only the walking, slowly, one foot in front of the other. If Hannah wanted to walk; Walk, we did. I was beside her every step of the way.

Each day, she meticulously chose clothes that were stylish. Scarves and swanky caps. She'd put some makeup on because it helped her feel brighter. She had turned twenty a few months before the radiation started. During this time, she had to scale back her uni studies to one unit. She wouldn't defer. It was her thread to normal and there was no way she was surrendering it, regardless of the physical and mental cost. Her study was her lifeline to a brilliant future.

In the heart of Sydney, the lack of green space was palpable. I ached to get my feet on soil. To be surrounded by and connected to nature in real time. I mentally rehearsed the feeling of being in my beloved bush back home, clear fresh air, no human-made sound within earshot, natural beauty of trees, wallabies, birds, insects and livestock. The closest space that wasn't covered by cement or tarmac was a small area of lawn and a few trees at the front of the Central Railway Station. I loved to go there and hangout with the trees and take a moment to pay my respects to a hearing guide dog called Donna. She was memorialised at the park with a plaque and monument.

Fitness was important to Hannah. We walked everywhere we could that was practical. We caught the train and Hannah loved to sit against the window. Most of the time, she would be asleep within a few minutes, gently leaning her head on my shoulder. It pained me to wake her when we got to our station in North Sydney. Then we had an arduous walk down a steep hill. The daily radiation became routine. The staff warmed to Hannah, and I think it broke their hearts to have this vibrant young twenty-year-old woman going through a hectic health experience. Most of the nurses were little older than her.

Nursing staff everywhere were amazing. They truly are our unsung heroes. Nurses and the staff that keep hospital wards functional make or break a hospital stay or treatment.

ride4acure ORIGIN STORY

The cleaners, ward helps and other hospital staff were always kind and compassionate. Everything and everyone mattered. They all were part of making those long months in and out of treatment and different hospitals bearable.

Chapter 10

Focus on What's Under Our Noses

We focused on the moment. None of us dwelt on the future, the 'what ifs' or prognoses. In fact, the only time Hannah ever asked about an outcome was when, months later, she was encouraged to try chemotherapy. It had a ridiculously low benefit for her. After being told by her new melanoma specialist that chemotherapy had lower than average outcomes for melanoma, She said, "Statistics are for average people, and I'm not average." None of us argued with that.

In the three months of the second round of treatment in Sydney, Hannah maintained a sense of positivity, humour, and kindness with those around her. I was awed daily by the inner strength that flowed from her. Never complaining, nor feeling sorry for herself or a skerrick of self-blame. She consistently found the light in every situation and put her focus there. She was pragmatic. Did what needed to be done, put her energy into giving it her best and being present.

I, on the other hand, at times let rip to the universe. I had definite moments of a strongly worded dialogue with God. My deep-seated sense of because I'd lived a life of service, generosity to community and family, I felt on some level, entitled to be blessed by not having shit things like this happening in my family. This belief was high on my complaints to God. Melanoma was a really shitty thing to happen to an unbelievably good and humble person like Hannah. I felt pissed off on her behalf. Many a time I had the 'enough already' conversation with God. I felt we had our limit of what we could deal with. How wrong I was.

Hannah was the reverse; she sailed through it. I never let her see my energy releases. I followed her lead on this one. It was her journey; I as her carer was in the wings.

I respected deeply all the health professionals Hannah dealt with. As a twenty-year-old young woman, she was treated with respect and intelligence. She made her own health decisions and my job was to support her choice.

Halfway through the two months of radiation, Adrian Stephens, the priest at Christ Church Saint Laurence, offered to say a healing mass concelebrated with a Mauritian priest, Father Ron. Hannah was moved by this offer and surrendered to the experience. She felt so supported and loved. She shared that though the 'one foot in front of the other' journey of treatment was tough, she genuinely felt her spirit was strong and powered by love.

Hannah was a beacon for us all on how to live life. In the depths of the lows, she found and focused on positives in her life. While her body was burnt to the core, she reflected on what would help her to return to health.

I realised some profound home truths during this time. The foundations for life in Hannah were strong. She wasn't focused on being someone for others, she focused on loving herself as she was. Hannah was loved by many. She was a person who was easy to love. Gentle, caring, witty, funny, intelligent, and capable. The two areas where her toughness came out were training horses and dogs. She was firm but fair with animals and gave them strong boundaries to relax into. She was unafraid to apply pressure when needed. With humans, she did that with subtly.

In our twenty years of our mum and daughter journey we never fought. Never raised our voices to each other. In fact, I rarely had a cross word with any of my kids. Esther and Joe, to this day, we've rarely argued. It's not that we always agree on things, it's simply that we value our differences and respect each other. I know I have different opinions in politics and, in some ways, spirituality. Some things I share stretch how they perceive the world and our humanity in it. Each of my kids have respected my values and I theirs.

What I now know is, as for most teenagers and young adults, some of their behaviours went underground and now they're older I'm hearing some curly stories for the first time and I love them all the more for trusting me to know now.

The kids and I worked as a team. My work with Full Circle Horsemanship included them. They loved working with me and the horses when I wasn't teaching. On weekends, we participated in horse sports at Pony Club, Campdrafting, Rodeos and trail riding in the Upper Macleay. Our lives centred around horses and the bush. We were at our happiest doing all these activities. Our horses were an extension of our family. We had a string of dogs too that were part of the crew.

Chapter 11

Burnt to a Crisp and Free

Hannah somehow navigated the two month's of radiation, and I survived too. Darcy was on the scene when work allowed, however, he was adrift. It was difficult for him to see the love of his life in so much pain and discomfort and fading in the second half of this treatment. He was still working on a property out near Yass and came into Sydney on weekends when there was no treatment. I gave them heaps of space. By now, Hannah was sleeping most of the day. She would watch her dodgy DVD rom-coms and doze on and off.

She had a strong desire for fresh lychees and it was a great distraction to go to Paddy's Market in Haymarket only a five-minute walk from the Presbytery. Hannah would lovingly peel these little gems of sweet food and take delicate nibbles, enjoying every morsel. I grew to love the relationship she had with lychees. They reminded her of the promise of life. To peel away an unsightly skin to reveal translucent deliciousness. Hannah lost her appetite and the only food she tolerated was soup and lychees.

The days blurred. Personal care, Hannah's radiation. Set and repeat.

Once the radiation was complete, Hannah and Darcy headed off. Darcy took Hannah to Queensland to meet his mum and dad.

On their return journey they called in and stayed with us for a few days at Temagog. It was a relief to spend ordinary time together outside a medical setting. In passing, Hannah mentioned a few times she was wondering how the little Jack Russell puppy had settled in to his new home? I had the breeder's phone number and on the quiet gave her a call. I was surprised to hear that she still had that one pup. The new owner at the last minute had been unable to take the pup and the breeder had decided to keep him. I shared with her that Hannah frequently asked about him and would she sell him? She agreed and I arranged to pick him up that afternoon. I sneakily told Hannah that we we're going to do a girl's trip to a new café and we left.

Burnt to a Crisp and Free

When I drove into the farm, the woman came walking toward our car with the pup trotting alongside her. Hannah burst into tears and jumped out of the car before I had barely stopped. She was overwhelmed to see and hold the pup and couldn't believe that he was hers now. The pup settled immediately on her shoulder, nestled into her neck. Hannah already had a name picked out, Hamish. She said every day since meeting him at Nana Glen the first time, she remembered the feeling of him laying on her neck and how happy he made her heart feel. In her mind she had already called him Hamish since the first moment they met.

As soon as she could, she was back to Charlton and working and studying again. She was doing distance learning now and working full time for Elders Pastoral Company at their Charlton Feedlot. She loved this work and the staff there. She was living with Darcy on a property just out of town near the racecourse at Charlton with friends of our family that go back a couple of generations through droving and mustering in Western NSW.

Hannah jammed as much life into the next few months as she could. Life was looking sweet for her. Work, study, love of her life, rodeoing and competing on her best mare Lena. Life was sweet.

I was back at work for TAFE NSW running horsemanship programs for at-risk young people and mature-aged students. I ran station hand courses and a Jillaroo school. Life was good and rich.

ride4acure ORIGIN STORY

As often as I could, I would do professional development with my horsemanship and attend training days. I was interested in a non-invasive equine technique to support muscle health for horses and had booked in to attend in the Hunter Valley. I took my horse Wrangler with me and we were on Day 2 or 3 when I got a call from Hannah. I was in my swag in the horse float, unable to sleep. It was late, nearly midnight, when my phone rang.

I answered, it was Hannah, and she said for the first time to me, "I don't feel well Mum."

In that moment, I had a stony cold feeling in the pit of my gut and a chill in every bone of my body.

"My back is killing me. Darcy took me into hospital, and they've given me Panadol and sent me home. Mum, I'm in pain. Bad pain." She almost whimpered.

I was over a thousand kilometres from Hannah. She was now in Western Victoria. Closest family was Melbourne, three hours away.

"Hannah, let me call an ambulance for you." I suggested.

"No Mum, don't do that!" she stated emphatically. "If you call it, I won't get in it. I'll be ok, I just need rest."

"Okay Han, I hear you, try to get some rest, I'll ring you in the morning sweetheart."

Burnt to a Crisp and Free

Our call ended.

I sat upright in my swag and breathed. I looked up into the crystal-clear night sky, littered with stars. I prayed.

"God, please help me, my daughter, bring the right people to help her now. Please help me stay strong and connected to you while we get through whatever's ahead."

I knew in my bones something was gravely wrong. I just didn't know exactly what.

I called my sister Kate, who lived in West Melbourne. She was a high school teacher and it was the middle of the night, around midnight. As soon as she picked up, I cried to her. I told her that Hannah wouldn't get in an ambulance and the 'take a Panadol' suggestion from the hospital. The cracker in that story was Hannah had told them about her melanoma journey and the recent months of radiation. She asked if it could be related to melanoma and they said no.

I was angry and scared to my core that melanoma was back. The plan I worked out with Kate was for her to drive to Charlton and go to Hannah. That was it. She would offer to take her to Melbourne to be checked and get some scans done.

Kate left immediately in her little purple Corolla, belting through the quiet country roads to Charlton. Three hours later, she knocked on Hannah's door and Hannah answered.

When she saw Kate standing there not saying anything, she said, "Mum sent you didn't she?"

She didn't want to pack an overnight bag and struggled out to Kate's car. Her back was killing her. She was wrapped in a fluffy blanket with the seat laid right back and they made their way back to Melbourne.

Sunrise saw them pulling into the hospital Emergency Department in Melbourne.

Kate has a way of making things happen and, as luck would have it, a brilliant, compassionate doctor triaged Hannah.

I was in Melbourne by midday that day and went straight to the hospital to Hannah and Kate.

The x-rays showed Hannah's liver was peppered with metastatic melanoma. The film looked like someone had emptied a money box of five cent pieces into it. Dark dots throughout. The news was devastating. Stage 4 metastatic melanoma.

Hearing this, my head filled with a rushing sound and everything receded. I felt like I was in a vortex.

In a twenty-year-old healthy girl who a few days before was happily riding her horses, working at the feedlot and using her brain to write brilliant essays, she was living the dream to become a livestock scientist with a passion for genetics.

How could my girl, for the third time in one short year, be on this roller coaster again?

I used all my inner power to be present to the people in the room.

The good news was Hannah met the most incredible medical person on the planet. Professor Grant McArthur. Her new melanoma specialist was so human. He oozed empathy and compassion with Hannah. Grant communicated with her at a deep level and told her everything she needed to know based on her questions. As always, it was Hannah's journey, and she led the dialogue. I wanted her to feel empowered.

Grant told Hannah about a specialist youth cancer service. No more getting shuffled between pillar and post for treatment. It was a one-stop patient-centred cancer service for young people based just up the road at the Peter Mac Cancer Centre.

Chapter 12

Another Universe

We had entered another universe. The staff were our angels with flesh on. Grant spent an hour sitting on the side of her bed, with me in the visitor's chair on that first consult. He carefully stepped her through every detail and then the treatment options. He asked about her life and was curious about her uni study and her passion for livestock science. He was young. Early forties, blond and light build. He a bit like Hannah's dad, Lindsay. Built like a greyhound, a compact powerhouse of energy.

We took exactly the same tack as we did in Sydney. This was Hannah's journey, and she was leading it. I was the support act as a carer. I felt in my bones to stand alongside her, be present, grounded, listen, hold the space. A million times I held back my 'Mum urge' to insist they do more and try more. I held my tongue over and over. The most important thread in the journey was for Hannah to feel empowered to make her own decisions. So much of her life was out of her hands. I trusted Hannah's creative mind to work through, use me as a sounding board and come back to making her own mind up about what she said yes to. Her new doctor Grant, was aligned fully with that approach, as was all the staff on the youth ward.

During triage at the first consult in Melbourne, it was explained to Hannah that if she stayed and didn't return to Sydney to her previous treatment team, what her options were. The grace of being in one spot with all the services she'd need being wrapped around her in one place was incredible. Peter Mac was a godsend.

The complexity of a scattered service model is a minefield to navigate. Navigate we did as we had no option the first two times. Once Hannah was under care in Peter Mac, Melbourne, it was the most incredible model of patient-centred care. The supports and services centred around her. Hannah was totally clear she wanted to stay in Victoria. There were a lot of family around, and it's where her horses were and, of course, Darcy.

Within a couple of days, Hannah had a team. Every thread of her life was attended to. It was a huge relief for me, as I was beyond capacity. Within days, Hannah was connected

Another Universe

to a brilliant social worker who helped her work through providing a health update to the University of New England and, best of all providing, a music therapist who created and played soft soulful music live to Hannah while they talked. They created a playlist of tracks that inspired, calmed and soothed, which Hannah loved to listen to.

When Hannah started chemo, a kind older woman who was a massage therapist came and gave her hand and foot massages. Hannah could be an outpatient with daily community nurse checks and visits to the hospital for treatment and chemo as needed. Strict instructions were given so if there were episodes of out-of-control pain again that couldn't be managed at home, to call an ambulance and come straight in.

Chapter 13

Trying for Normal

I was in touch with Hannah's line manager from the Elders Feedlot at Charlton.

She was so supportive and genuinely loved Hannah, and shared with me plans the company had to support Hannah to work and study. She said her company recognised talent and wanted to nurture that. Hannah at this stage was halfway through her Livestock Science degree and still unbelievably studying. She'd reduced her study workload while she navigated this round of treatment.

It was such a privilege to be surrounded by a circle of people who all had Hannah's best interests at heart as well as so many family members and friends visit her.

ride4acure ORIGIN STORY

We'd been at Kate's for about a week. Kate lived in West Melbourne in a terrace house with her twin daughters, Sarah and Liz, who were nineteen and navigating uni and work. It was a two-bedroom long and narrow building. Kate had a tiny front yard which she'd filled with plants. A long passage from the front door, with two bedrooms on the left. The passage led down into the living area, a lounge room, dining room and small kitchen. The toilet was about fifteen metres to the furthest corner of the backyard, which meant walking along a narrow path through more gardens, and past her small chook pen with four red hens in it.

It was a vibrant little green space in the backyard with an outdoor table under grapevines. This area was so peaceful to sit in and relax. Hannah and I spent quite a bit of our time on sunny days out there relaxing, playing cards and talking.

Esther was pre-training race horses in Port Macquarie and was in a share house with a couple of jockeys and a farrier. When we landed in Melbourne, she immediately came to be with us. She got a job riding track work at Flemington close to Kate's and was gone at 4 am each morning for about five hours. When she'd come back, she would lie beside Hannah while she still smelt of horses and tell her every detail of each horse she rode. Hannah would close her eyes and breathe it all in, every little detail. My heart melted seeing my two girls side by side sharing stories. It had been their way for eighteen years. They were joined at the hip. For life. This was their love language. Tangled limbs, shared breath, horse stories. So much of their story didn't have words, it simply was.

Trying for Normal

Joe was flown from Kempsey to Melbourne as an unaccompanied minor with Qantas. He was only ten years old. It was tough for Joe, as all my attention was with Hannah and he was on the sideline. Each of the three times that year Hannah had to have Joe come to spend time with her, it was a lot of unknown for him to be close to. This time though, he needed to be with us.

Here was this monumental experience Hannah was having and Esther, Joe, Lindsay and I were all trying to stay focused on the future. A future where Hannah was well, thriving and living a great life. Hannah was busy scheduling how she would finish her degree, her work and dreaming into the potential USA opportunity and what it meant to be in love with Darcy. Darcy kept moving between Charlton and Melbourne and visited as often as he could.

Her doctor had arranged for community nursing to come to Hannah at Kate's home to check her daily and monitor pain. It was such a terrific arrangement, as it meant no navigating traffic to get to the hospital. It was patient-centred care a hundred percent. Everything was about what's best for Hannah.

To sleep, Hannah and I shared a pull-out sofa bed in the lounge, which meant when Kate and the girls needed to go to any part of the house, they had to walk through the space. We were grateful for Kate and the girl's generosity to have us there while Hannah wasn't an inpatient, however, it wasn't conducive to rest, but it was the best we had.

ride4acure ORIGIN STORY

On about day four of staying at Kate's, I woke in the middle of the night, pitch dark and eerily quiet, to find Hannah not in the bed with me. I reached across and felt her side of the sofa bed and it was cold. I knew she'd been gone for a while. I was dead to the world sleeping as I was exhausted.

On high alert, I leapt out of bed and rushed through the house and down out into the yard and could see the toilet light on. As I got closer, I could hear Hannah moaning and crying. I rushed to her. My beautiful girl was doubled over in agony. The pain was off the scale and she couldn't get off the loo. I breathed with her and she came through some of the pain, enough to find her feet with help and after a long, slow walk along the garden path, we got back inside the house, dosed her up on pain medication and got her back to bed.

I didn't sleep a wink after this. I was lying on my side listening to her precious breaths going in and out of her body. As a mother, my fierce protectiveness is at the forefront. This moment galvanised this for me; we needed a better plan. Hannah didn't want to be an inpatient, but this wasn't working for us. Hannah and I loved being with family, but our days of living in a heritage terrace house with an outdoor loo were over from that moment.

Each time I'd checked in with Hannah's boss, she'd said, "Please let me know if there's anything you need."

Trying for Normal

The next day, I phoned and told her what had happened describing the situation we were in. At this point I was living on carer's leave which was rapidly dwindling. This was the fourth round of medical events in eleven months. I was broke. I didn't have the money to rent a place close to the city for Hannah's treatment. I put my 'big girl pants on' and asked straight out if the company would support us with accommodation. Her boss didn't hesitate a nanosecond. She immediately said yes and then reassured me she would organise everything. Within twenty-four hours, we were in a ground floor open-plan apartment with the most comfortable king-sized bed we'd ever slept in and a luxury bathroom, with a walk-in shower and an indoor toilet. A kitchen where we could cook and prepare nutritious food.

Hannah had been on wheat grass juice. I'd found a provider who home delivered, and we had a tray of fresh wheatgrass every couple of days. Hannah and all of us were living on a fresh food, nutrition-dense diet. We all thrived. My sister Veronica, who Hannah had a close relationship with, came to stay for a few days. It all felt so normal. We were tuned into a 'we've got this' feel. We had ten days living like this and it was blissful. Hannah perked up immensely. Her pain meds got changed, and that helped. Lindsay came to Melbourne from Ivanhoe to be with Hannah.

The South Melbourne apartment felt like a turning point. We had a week and a bit where it truly felt that things were on the up. Hannah's energy was increasing and her pain was decreasing. She had started chemo and there was great hope it would slow down the metastasising of the tumours, of which there were many scattered through her liver. Hannah was taking a comprehensive cocktail of medications. I was administering morphine and pain meds through a port in her tummy. We had community nurses visit daily to check in.

The model and quality of care was incredible. We truly felt like things were turning the corner. Hannah was responding and feeling on the up. Joe, Esther, Lindsay and I were with Hannah watching movies; other family members came and went. Her favourite movies were Kung Fu Panda and the full box set of Kath and Kim. Hannah's appetite was increasing a little, and we celebrated with her favourite foods. She had only bite-sized tastes and savoured every morsel. She wrote lists and plans for how her life was going to pan out. One month, three months, semesters and years from this moment. She mapped how she'd catch up and finish her degree. Her dream to go to America and work. Plans for her and Darcy. List after list of 'seeds of the paths' her life may take.

On day ten of chemo, I was alone with Hannah when she had another bout of excruciating pain that caused her to nearly black out. We were under strict instructions that if the pain got worse, to call an ambulance immediately. I did. I was terrified to see her in so much pain. The threshold kept increasing. Within minutes, we were in an ambulance on the way to the hospital.

Trying for Normal

At hospital Grant met Hannah and examined her fully. He suggested she stay in the hospital in the youth ward so he could monitor her. I agreed wholeheartedly. It was terrifying as a carer to have now supported Hannah through two episodes of out-of-control pain. Even with all the support, I couldn't nurse her at home anymore. It was too much. I was terrified and relieved.

This was not like any other hospital we'd been in. Every consideration was given to us to enable the best experience for the patient and us as family.

PeterMac arranged accommodation for the rest of my family right beside the hospital, only a two-minute walk to Hannah's hospital room. Her cousins started coming and her girlfriends from Kempsey arrived in a steady stream. I stayed in Hannah's room with her and had a stretcher set up.

Amanda, one of Hannah's cousins, was bringing Hannah's Jack Russell dog Hamish into the hospital in a large shoulder bag so Hannah could have a cuddle. Hamish would snuggle in alongside her in bed and pump his love vibes into her body. It was one of my, 'better to ask for forgiveness than permission' moments. I'm sure the staff knew, but no one had the heart to stop us.

Hannah could no longer walk. To go to the loo, she had to get in a wheelchair and I'd wheel her in. Each time we went into the ensuite bathroom she commented the mirror was too high. If she was designing a bathroom, she'd have it so patients in wheelchairs could see their faces. It made me smile that there she was thinking about others and wanting them to have a better experience.

Hannah progressively declined, and it was clear things were not going where we wanted. However, the word 'death' was never mentioned because in my mind, I didn't think she would die. I simply couldn't fathom that she could and the thought didn't arise. I held on to the miniscule hope of a miracle. I had a prayer tree extending across the country.

As it was the week before Christmas, the ward was nearly empty of other patients. I spent time talking to the other young people. Many of whom were alone. No family except for a short visit now and again. It pained me. Here was Hannah with dozens of family and friends, many of whom flew on short notice from out of state and her home town of Kempsey to visit.

Hannah had asked Grant about why young people got melanoma. He patiently sat with her and described in detail the why of melanoma and that predominantly it was caused through UV exposure by the sun. And that eighty percent of skin cell damage happens before we're 18 years old. Sometimes it's a genetic thing, but most of the time it's sun damage.

Hannah asked if there was a clinical trial somewhere in Australia or the world, she could be a part of and he said, "Sadly not."

Trying for Normal

"Why not?" asked Hannah.

"Because at this time, there's not the research dollars, Hannah, for this disease," he said.

We all sat in silence at that. The enormity of those words sinking in for all of us. *No clinical trial anywhere in the world.*

Hannah turned to me and with her face lit up and her eyes locked in mine said, "Mum, when we get through this thing, you and I are going to do something to raise money to help Grant find a cure!" I reached out and held her hand and promised her we would.

Even with all the evidence under my eyes, I stubbornly held onto hope. Not one person around me mentioned Hannah dying to my face or to her. Her focus, like mine, was on recovery. She had so much life to live. We were relentlessly optimistic.

After a week in hospital, the daily decline of Hannah's capacity to move, eat, speak, and stay conscious decreased before my eyes. Grant came in and sat on Hannah's bed. He said, "Hannah, there's no more treatment left we can use for you. Our goal now is to manage your pain with medication."

The tumours had spread further. The pain Hannah was in at times was unbelievable. New depths of agony unfolded daily. Hannah was required to have an MRI and needed to go in the tunnel. To do that required her to lie flat. I was beside her as they prepared her to go in. She couldn't lay flat. In her hospital bed she'd been propped on pillows, with her mattress inclined to take pressure off and relieve the pain. It was agony for her to lie flat and the nurses tried to be understanding but were insistent. I was begging them to not do the scan. Couldn't they see how impossible it was? I felt deeply distressed. Hannah began groaning, and it took me back to the ward in Sydney after round two of surgery and the older women groaning in their beds. I felt such deep desolation and helplessness wash over me.

Powerless to take an iota of pain from my beautiful girl in her deep need, I was begging God to give me the pain to bear, to relieve her of this burden. I would've a thousand times over laid my life down to take her pain away. I have never felt so helpless in my life. Ever. I knew at that moment this was it. There was no coming back from this. With all the medication in the world for pain, nothing was touching the agony she was in. After that intervention, the pain increased yet again and the new drugs administered meant she was unconscious a lot more. We were told probably wouldn't be lucid as much but would be much more comfortable.

Many an hour I begged God to heal Hannah, that I would take this burden if it had to be borne by someone, but to heal Hannah. I petitioned relentlessly and had many others doing the same, praying for healing. By this stage, it was inevitable that Hannah's moments on earth were dwindling.

Trying for Normal

Time slowed to a pulse for me. Every breath, every pulse, every heartbeat was a precious gift. Sadly, one which I had taken for granted. As mother to three incredible kids, to bear witness to my eldest slowly preparing to leave earth was beyond me. But bear witness, I did. Those last three or so days, I didn't close my eyes. I didn't want to miss a moment with her. Day and night, I was with her. By her side.

Sometimes the pain medication didn't hit the spot for Hannah and she was in agony. I would position myself at the foot of the bed and gently hold my hands over the arches of her feet and she would slowly change from moaning in agony to peaceful relaxation. I didn't know why I went to her feet the first time. I simply felt what to do and that was what came to me. From the moment I laid my hands over her arches, she settled and would drift into a peaceful place. Whatever was happening energetically between us calmed her and brought her peace. If during these times I took my hands more than an inch from her arches, the pain would return. I stood at her feet in vigil, endlessly for hours.

I would've sacrificed anything in myself to keep Hannah breathing. That was and is my truth.

The death knoll had been rung. Melanoma was raging out of control and it was inevitable that death was the outcome.

A switch went in my mind. If the hours and minutes were all she had, every single second was going to count.

ride4acure ORIGIN STORY

I asked Hannah if she could have anyone visit her who would it be and she said, "Lena". Her magnificent palomino mare.

Bec, her cousin who was in Charlton, a three-hour drive away, flew into action and brought Lena into Melbourne to Fitzroy Gardens next to the hospital early the next day. The hospital is in the centre of Melbourne, right near St Patrick's Cathedral.

On a sublime summer's day, Darcy, with Esther, pushed the bed with Hannah propped up in it, giggling as they went. It was a major production to navigate the bed out of the hospital, down the footpath, across Lansdowne Street, into the park.

Hannah had six pillows under her upper body to keep her in the least painful position with her body. She was so serene. She spent time doing her hair, then put a cap on it. I had to manage the pillows. She would ask me lovingly to fluff the pillows and told everyone that I knew exactly how to fluff them. There was a running joke about Mum's magic pillow fluffing. Hannah was like our princess propped up on her bed, with Hamish, her dog, happily sitting onboard with her. She was happy and aminated. Lindsay, her dad, Darcy, and Esther were in charge of steering the bed. Aunty Veronica and I took turns pushing each other in the wheelchair, giggling like schoolgirls. To cross the street, a few of us were on traffic control and did an unofficial traffic stop to get the bed across Lansdowne Street and into the park.

Trying for Normal

Hannah relished being outside after eight days inside. She was a few floors from ground level. A million miles from her beloved bush environment. Hannah had an energy boost anticipating seeing her animals and to have so many of our family around her for a few hours in a green outdoor space like Fitzroy Gardens. Huge towering elm trees, with paths meandering through the perfectly manicured lawns.

Not long after we got settled in the park in a patch of sunshine, we got the phone call to say Lena was only a few blocks away. Hannah's cousin Rebecca and one of the girls from the feedlot were in the ute with precious Lena in the float. Hannah perked up and was so excited to see Lena's rump over the tailgate of the horse float. The driver simply 'jumped' the gutter with the float and pulled the ute and float up in the gardens. Hannah insisted she be right at the float to make sure Lena was unloaded safely. As soon as Lena was backed out and came straight to Hannah and lowered her head. She breathed out audibly over Hannah's heart, then did long sweeps up and down her body from head to toe. She then rested her muzzle over Hannah's belly so Hannah could touch her. Hannah kept saying, "My beautiful mare. My little champ."

There wasn't a dry eye amongst us. It was plain for us all to see was the bond and love between this young woman and her mare. A deep gratitude expressed in the gentle stroking of Hannah's hand down Lena's forehead and muzzle. A lifetime of rides that wouldn't be had. Their journey was at an end.

For all of us surrounding Hannah who were horsemen and women, this was an ineffable moment. Beyond words and understanding. Our hearts knew what was going on, and they were breaking. All of us crying. After a few minutes, the moment was broken when Lena lifted her head and Hannah asked Kate for Lena's snacks. She had asked Aunty Kate to prepare well cut-up snacks of apple and carrots for Lena. They had to be cut up small, as according to Hannah, "Lena doesn't like chunky bits."

Kate dutifully prepared a container of horse snacks that Hannah lovingly fed to Lena who reciprocated by dribbling apple and carrot slobber all over Hannah which made her laugh and giggle. It was all love for Hannah. Her mare, her dogs, Hamish and Bobby, family and friends. Throughout this last week, she would often raise her hand and gently touch my cheek and say, "Do you know how much I love you, Mum?"

"To the moon and back Hannah, I know, and I love you," I responded each time with tears flowing unbidden down my cheeks.

In Fitzroy gardens, Darcy was so attentive to Hannah. We created a love nest of pillows and cushions, at the base of the trunk of an ancient English Elm tree for them and gently Lindsay and Esther lifted her into a comfy position alongside Darcy so she could lean against him and the tree and have a snuggle. Hannah was still holding Lena's lead rope and the mare never once put pressure on it as she

Trying for Normal

grazed the sweet mown Fitzroy Gardens manicured lawn. The mare knew her human needed her to be close. They stayed there for an hour or so and we all wandered off and gave them space.

A white official-looking work ute came at some speed across the gardens and I quickly walked away from my gathering toward them. The driver launched out of the ute quite furious however I held my hand up and said, "Look over there mate, my daughter is dying and she wanted to say goodbye to her horse and us her family outside."

The man changed in an instant and was visibly moved by what he was witnessing; he choked up holding back his own tears. In that moment I knew he was envisioning himself and his own kids in that situation. I promised to pick up any horse poo and leave no trace of where we'd been. They quietly drove away from what was possibly a first for him to witness.

Veronica and I had wheelchair races along the paths, avoiding collisions with a few trees. We were screaming and laughing like little girls without a care in the world. No one would guess that fifty metres away, my daughter was preparing to leave earth.

I relished in those moments of freedom, laughter and delight. For a few short minutes, I was simply present in this garden, my big; boisterous family, who showed up when it mattered most. To bear witness with me as we companioned one of us that was dying.

ride4acure ORIGIN STORY

We stayed there until Hannah let us know it was time we went back. We packed up all the picnic things. Hannah was gently placed back on her bed and Lena came to her and Hannah and Lena rested their foreheads together.

The tears flowed freely in all of us, witnessing the most incredible moments between these two. Human and horse. We could again hear Lena audibly breathe on Hannah.

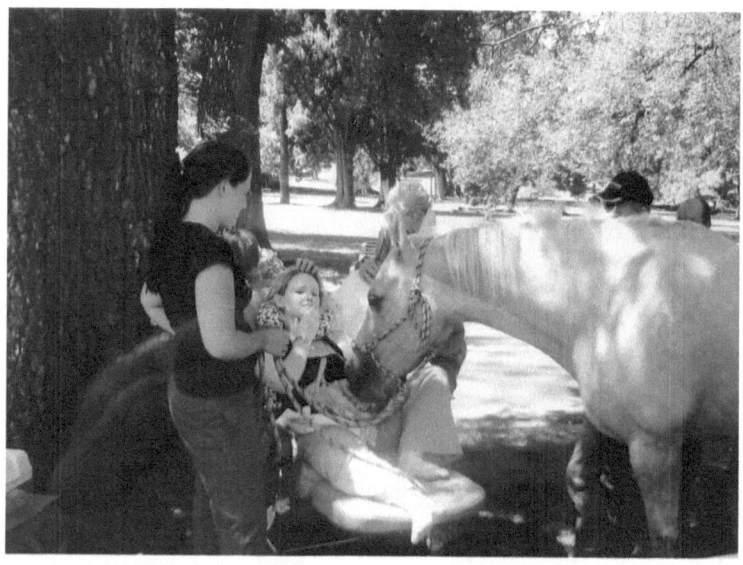

**Final goodbyes Hannah and Lena
Fitzroy Gardens Melbourne Vic**

Trying for Normal

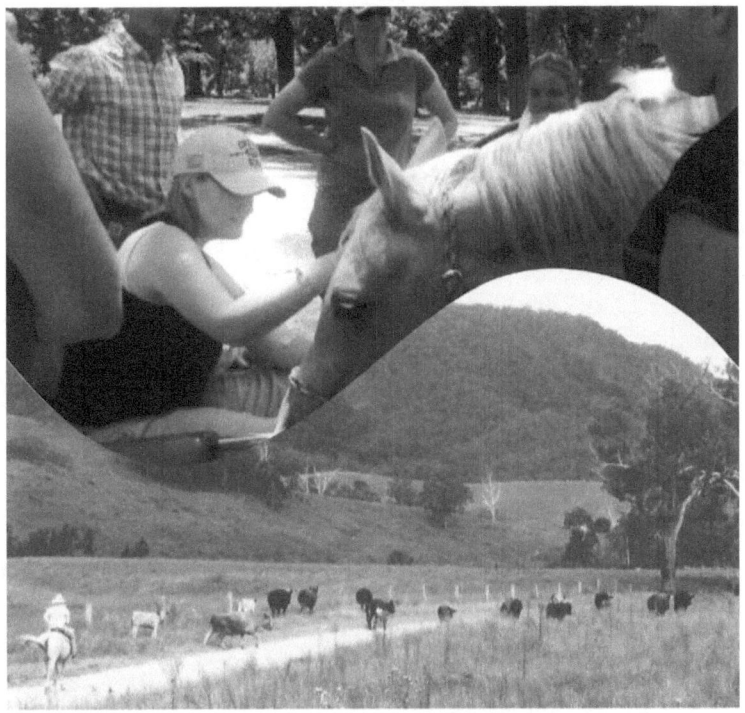

Top: Fitzroy Gardens, the day before Hannah left earth.
Final goodbye Hannah & Lena.
Bottom: Remembering Hannah's happy
place, Moparrabah farm life.

Lena was loaded back in the float under Hannah's careful eye. My feet were heavy returning. I slowly walked the several hundred metres back to the hospital. Every step was never to be repeated. Each step closer to the hospital was one less, never-to-be-repeated moment with Hannah.

My heart was buoyant and heavy at the same time. Rivers of tears poured from me daily in the quiet moments, unwitnessed by others. As I had watched the ute and float disappear from my view, I knew that Lena and Hannah's journey together on earth was complete, just as mine soon would be as her mother on earth. I knew our bond was stronger than earthbound. The thought of never touching, seeing, speaking to Hannah again was creeping into my cells. It awoke a conviction in me to double down on taking emotional snapshots of all these moments, to savour in the times ahead.

I drank in the softness of her skin, her serene blue eyes that were pools of wonder. Hannah had breathed in the mysteries and secrets her whole life. She saw things hidden to most. Many a time, as little girls, Hannah and Esther would have a game with their animals, and there would always be fairies and angels thrown in, watching over them.

I let the men push Hannah's bed back to hospital and walked slowly at the rear of the family procession back toward the hospital. My sister Veronica walked with me and put her arm around my shoulders and held me close as we slowly walked, one foot in front of the other. She knew this path intimately as she'd lost her boy Max when he was only nine. It became one more thing Veronica and I shared. A title that neither of us wanted. Bereaved mothers.

As I stepped through the automatic doors into the hospital, I caught the lift back up to Hannah's room. Veronica and I lovingly showered her and then we got her back in bed. We did as much of the nursing ourselves as we wanted hands of love to be remembered by Hannah. The nurses were brilliant, but we wanted to care for her as much as possible.

One thing that struck me was the life pouring in and out of Hannah. She was when animated, bright and engaging. The couple of other young people on the ward were mostly alone, with the odd visitor coming for a few minutes. These young people walked around with the weight of the world on their shoulders. My heart broke for them as they looked like the walking dead with nothing to live for. Here was our Hannah, full of life, as she was dying with a brilliant life to live for, but that wasn't to be her journey. Her time earth-side was coming to an end.

At one stage Lindsay and I were standing on either side of Hannah's bed, talking across it. Hannah was in a deep sleep. Though the staff had said she would most likely not be conscious with the new medication, she was a lot of the time.

Lindsay's sister Sandi was on her way from Wangaratta to say goodbye and Lindsay and I were trying through our tired brains to remember her husband's name. We both knew it well, but in that moment were drawing blanks. We went back and forth with options for a few minutes, then Hannah, without opening an eye, said to us both quite loudly, "It's Mick ya dickheads!"

We were shocked to silence and then both laughed out loud because she was right. Shocked because she'd called us both dickheads, which she'd never done in her twenty years. And then laughing out loud as it was hilarious.

After the surgery in Sydney in September, Hannah had lost nerves that affected on her capacity to raise her arm higher than her shoulder. During these last few days, she would reach upwards with that arm, with no limitation. Her hand was extended as if reaching for someone's hand.

Father Michael Smith, who is a family friend and Jesuit priest, came to visit Hannah and anointed her with Holy Oils for her final voyage. It was a heartfelt ritual with just Lindsay, Esther, and Joe in the room with Hannah, Father Michael, and I. This ritual amplified the connection with all those who had passed before us. Many a time in those last few days, I said to Fr Michael that 'the room was crowded'. I could feel the presence of Mum, Dad, Grandma, my nephew Maxie and my good mate Ginger who had died in 1986. They were all there waiting for her. This 'crossing over' and the connection to family on the other side gave me great comfort. Don't get me wrong, I wanted to keep her earthside more than anything. This was a little balm for my soul. The veil between the worlds is thin. The sense of safety and comfort on 'the other side' was palpable for me in those last 24 hours. I could feel the energy of companions in the room awaiting her.

Hannah's girlfriend circle from her St Paul's School days had come to see her in Melbourne, several of their mums too. Those precious school years where our families blended.

Trying for Normal

It was such a comfort to have these girls who had been like sisters. It brought so much joy to Hannah that they were present. There was a lot of resting of hands. That peace-giving signal of simply resting a hand on an arm or the back of a hand or holding hands.

The beauty in these moments brought me to tears. The preciousness of physical touch and knowing this soul will soon be out of physical touch with each of us.

I watched Hannah's energy closely as people came and went. Hannah was drifting in and out of consciousness. However, she still maintained a sense of presence as witnessed in her 'It's Mick ya dickheads' statement.

I never left the room and as each person came in, I watched Hannah's energy. Often, she would unconsciously, like a gentle wave, move toward the person's energy as they entered and would visibly relax. For a few tricky people on entry, she quickly jerked away. Veronica and I were the guardians at the gate and would usher those people quickly back out of the room. It wasn't their time to be with Hannah. She needed peace. Time was too precious. Every nanosecond counted.

I asked Hannah what she felt like for dinner that night. She was barely eating. Tiny morsels; however she was keenly interested in what others were having. This night she asked for a lamb kebab. There was a ripper kebab shop a few blocks away, so Darcy and a few others were on a mission for this sacred lamb kebab. In companionship with her, we all had exactly the same kebab as her, lamb, with all the salads and garlic aioli.

We sat together in her room, every space taken up on the floor, her bed. The stretcher had bodies on it. We were all savouring the taste and sharing of what would most likely be our last meal together. We'd propped her up on her pillows as comfortable as she could be in readiness for this meal. There were about a dozen of her closest family and friends in the room. She was as alert as she'd been down in Fitzroy Gardens with Lena. Chatty, funny, cracking jokes, she'd begin telling stories and then drift off and allow someone else to take over the telling. The feeling in the room was so rich and loving. I drank it in. This young life, such good staunch friends and family who loved her deeply. The DVD her friends made played out on a loop with pictures of her life beamed up on the wall so she could see it became the prompt for many of the stories.

Grant McArthur and the nursing staff were amazed at how those days played out for us. Grant would often come in and sit with us.

"You know how to do caring. This is perfect, everything your doing is perfect," he'd say.

Not once was the word palliative care used. I didn't really know what it was at that stage however I now know; it was what we were doing. Bringing as much life as possible to these simple moments, that became hours, that became the rest of her life.

Hannah held her lamb kebab and looked dreamily at it. I thought about the simple acts in life, like eating a kebab and how prior to this moment I would've taken it for granted. This moment of Hannah not fully knowing, but suspecting, this would be the last thing she would taste as a human and share with many of the people who she loved most in the world, made that moment count. She looked at that kebab like it was the love of her life. She breathed in the rich aromas of the roast meat, the hummus, garlic aioli. She took the tiniest nibble of meat and savoured it for minutes with her eyes closed. I felt she was memorising the taste. A tiny bite of the cool, crunchy lettuce, relishing the creamy richness of cheese. This choice of meal was in contrast to what Hannah had been eating, only having sips of soups, and her beloved fresh lychees for weeks.

That night was such an experience of solidarity. All of us chowing down on our lamb kebabs with Hannah like there would be a thousand more moments like this. The room was full of chatter, laughter, and yarns being shared. We had about three visitor chairs in the room and my fold out stretcher, which had four people sitting on it. The rest were on the floor, a few of us sitting on the bed. One wall playing the constant loop of moments of shared life with Hannah. It was perfect. Hannah was soaking up her life's moments. We were marinating in hers.

Most of my family that had travelled to be in Melbourne were staying next door to the hospital in the hospital accommodation or at Kate's place in West Melbourne. Lindsay, Esther, and Joe were all next door. Veronica and her family. Liz had travelled down from Boree Creek. Liz had a close relationship with Hannah, having a couple of times during her own young adult life come and stayed with us for a period of time.

Hannah slept peacefully that night. Darcy was there and helped me get her ready for bed. I gave them time alone for ten minutes, but then Hannah called me back in to fluff her pillows. I made a nest for her to rest and stroked her cheek. She reciprocated and again repeated lovingly, "You know how much I love you, Mum?"

And I responded I did with all my heart and that I'd loved her first. I'd loved her from the moment I knew she was within me. And that won't change.

She drifted into a deep sleep. The next morning, Fr Michael came in to pray. We stood around her bed. I was beside Hannah but looking straight out the window into the cityscape over the rooftops. Suddenly I saw three large white birds in formation flying right to the window. I gasped sharply as I thought they would break the glass, but at the last minute they changed course and flew upwards and I saw their bellies. I heard the words, "We're Hannah's angels and we've come to carry her out of here." Not long after this, Hannah desperately asked me, "Mum, mum, how will I get off earth?"

I leant down close to her and whispered, "Hannah there is a chorus of angels coming to carry you out of here."

She laid back in her bed and said with a smile on her face, "That's okay, then."

With that she reached upward with her semi-paralysed arm, hand outstretched as if reaching for someone's hand, still smiling took a full inhale of breath that was to be her last, and at 10.10am left earth, carried peacefully away with her three angels.

I noted the time and quietly cried and smiled at the same time, as I knew it was a sign. Hannah died at the same time she was born, 10.10am. It meant something to me and me alone. It wasn't a random act. There was a pattern in this. Lindsay and I clung to each other in that moment, sobbing together, holding each other beside our girl. Our beautiful girl that we'd lovingly bought into the world had left. Esther and Joe, huddled in. The nurse came in after a few minutes and declared Hannah dead.

Fr Michael and I stayed and prayed together. My hands resting gently on Hannah's hand and shoulder.

After about forty minutes, I realised for the first time that it was the 22nd of December, three days before Christmas. I had been so focused on having family close at every stage of her journey with melanoma that I knew with every cell of my being that Hannah needed to be buried before Christmas.

She wasn't going to a morgue. Her body couldn't be on her own, away from us her loved ones. We needed to stay together until she was laid to rest in her mother the earth.

The manager in me took over. Alone in the room with Hannah, I fell to my knees and prayed.

"God, I need a miracle. It's three days before Christmas. I need to keep Hannah with me in this circle of love until she's laid to rest in the earth. Help me. I can't do this alone."

I stood up, picked up my phone and called the funeral directors who had arranged both Mum and Dad's funerals. I asked to speak to the senior person that had a soft spot for us Luxfords.

By some miracle, she picked the phone up on the first ring.

"'Hi, its Maura Luxford, Marie and Kevin's daughter. Long story short, my daughter Hannah has died this morning here in Melbourne." I gave her the sixty-second-wrap of the situation and how we'd cared for Hannah all the way through her treatment and that I couldn't bear the thought of her being in a morgue for weeks over Christmas.

"I need you to arrange a funeral for Gisborne Catholic Church before Christmas," I stated.

"Maura, that's impossible. It can't happen. It takes at least a week. And Maura, at this time of year, three days before

Trying for Normal

Christmas, it won't happen until new year. I simply can't do it." she gasped at me.

"I'm going to be straight up and down on this, I'm desperate, I'm not asking. I'm stating, to you and your team what we need. What I need. I need you to make this happen. Do whatever it takes. We need the funeral before Christmas. Hannah can't go to a morgue. She has to stay with us. Now, I'm going to end this call. I'm staying with Hannah until you ring me back with the details. And I need a plot facing trees near her cousin Max's grave at Gisborne. Please, please help us make this happen." Then I hung up.

I fell to my knees again; I prayed like I'd never prayed in my life. I saw in my mind's eye every detail coming together. The mass at the old church in Gisborne, a walking procession to the cemetery a kilometre up the road led by her mare Lena, covered in a garland of flowers. Time will stretch to allow us to make this happen. I told myself over and over that two days is all the time in the world we need for us to arrange the details to give Hannah her ceremony to leave earth.

I told everyone to act as if this was going to happen. In my mind and heart, there was no alternative. She wasn't going to a morgue to sit there for weeks over Christmas. That was final. I was determined. The energy that was alive in me at that moment was steel-like. With every fibre of my being, I knew what was needed. I'd been by Hannah's side for twelve months through this and no way was I leaving now until the earth received her.

I stayed on my own with Hannah, praying. I didn't entertain for a nanosecond Hannah going to the morgue and being apart from her body. There simply wasn't a thought in me that was separate to that reality. There was no 'what ifs'.

My family were incredible, and everyone worked together behind the scenes to make this possible.

Kate had set to work organising an industrial air conditioner so we could take Hannah's body back to her place to rest in the lounge room to be delivered that day.

Forty-five minutes later my phone rang; it was the funeral director. She said matter of factly, "How's 2pm on 24 December at Gisborne?"

That's when I cried hard. The torrents opened and through my tears I said, "Perfect, that's perfect, thank you, thank you."

She sounded pleased that her company had made this happen against all the odds.

I thanked her beyond my heart's capacity. I knew she'd come through. With that, we could transfer Hannah to Kate's place within a couple of hours. The air conditioner was organised, the room prepared by her cousins and Kate. Hannah came home with us until her funeral in two days' time.

Trying for Normal

Kate had made a receptive space in the lounge for her to be lain out with flowers and candles. There were chairs, stools around the space for people to sit and be with her.

Lindsay and Esther set about buying her new clothes for her to be buried in. A barrel racing shirt, her beloved jeans with fancy stitching on the pockets, and then dressed her, with her Fat Boy boots propped beside her feet. Esther and a few of the girls did her hair and makeup using some special diamond clips for her hair.

Father Adrian Stephens had given Hannah a colourful crucifix that was handmade from a Benedictine Abbey on her first day of radiation back in Sydney. Adrian had worn this crucifix himself as it was a favourite of his. However, one day when we were having breakfast together. "Hannah, do you have a crucifix?" Adrian asked gently.

"No," she said.

Adrian took the crucifix off his own neck and with so much love handed it to Hannah. Hannah kept that cross with her at every step of the journey, tucked in her pocket. Remembering the love and power of that moment I put it in her jeans pocket to go with her to heaven.

Joe drew drawings just for Hannah. He didn't show them to any of us. He folded them up and placed them in her jean pockets. Joe made sure she had a hair tie, and a strawberry flavoured lip smacker in her pockets too, and he proudly told us in his biggest ten-year-old voice that Hannah wouldn't go anywhere without those two things. He was right. He knew her.

We had two days to plan all the funeral arrangements and organise the plot next to Hannah's cousin Max in Gisborne cemetery. My brother Mick and his daughter Rebecca arranged for Lena, her mare, and Bobby and Hamish, her two dogs, to be present for the funeral.

I met at Kate's kitchen table with funeral directors and picked out a coffin and flowers, including a massive garland of roses that were to be placed on the coffin, then for Lena to wear from the church to the cemetery.

Sam, Hannah's cousin, organised a large photo of Hannah and Lena barrel racing to be on an easel at the front of the church.

The order of proceedings for the service was a delight. I picked readings. The cousins made their own prayers of the faithful, her cousins were to do the communion altar procession. As many family members and friends as possible were to be included in every step of the mass.

Amazingly, the details came together and fell into place.

Hannah was in prize position in the lounge room. We sat and told stories, drank tea and included her in these moments. I still was barely sleeping. My mind and heart bursting with grief at the reality that Hannah would soon be in the ground, out of sight and touch, however at the same time I was holding myself and being present to the myriad of tasks that needed doing.

These two precious days at Kate's were the balm we all needed to be present with the footprint, the journey with which Hannah had left in all our hearts.

Joe spent a lot of time drawing pictures and writing little stories and tucking them into Hannah's pockets. It was both heartening and heart breaking. Hannah was his ballast. His rock. She loved him with all her heart, and he knew it. Hannah could pull him into line in a second and he yielded. They had respect and a genuine love for each other.

A few years before, when we were still at the farm at Moparrabah, Hannah was about fifteen. She'd got a massive bucket of Malteser chocolates for her birthday. She shared them out one at a time to Esther and Joe, and then they were stored in her wardrobe. Hannah never gutsed food down, was always deliberate in the way she ate and stretched the sweet treats out to enjoy. About a week into the chocolates being in the house, Joe at six years old, couldn't contain himself and he found the bucket and ate the lot. Made himself sick and Hannah was furious with him, gave him a right old bawling out about stealing. From then on, if Joe was being sneaky about something, Hannah would simply say, "Malteser?" to remind Joe to be honest. Lesson learnt.

The thing about the way Hannah disciplined Joe was he never doubted she loved him. He took whatever punishment was doled out to him. She was fair, but firm most of the time. Sometimes when Joe was particularly annoying when Hannah had mates staying at the farm, she'd asked him politely a few times to cease whatever annoying behaviour he was demonstrating, then she would warn him to stop or he'd cop it.

She would say to him, "What do we do with dogs when they're annoying, Joe?"

"Tie them up," Joe would respond and she'd give him the side eye.

A few times Joe pushed it too far and she would quietly get up, silently frog march him outside while he was pleading with her that he was sorry and would stop. She'd get him out the back door and grab a lead rope off the hat rack and take him to a tree a few metres from the back verandah and tie him up, wrapping the rope round and round his body and tying behind the tree so he couldn't get to the knot. Slightly bordering on child abuse, however, within ten minutes he was as acquiescent as a dove and begging to be untied, yelling he'd do the right thing. Humiliating but effective behaviour management strategy for super annoying little brothers.

As we navigated the two days at Kate's, these memories were distant. All the focus was on the girl and young woman

Trying for Normal

she'd been in all our lives. Kind, compassionate, funny, intelligent, and generous. Our lives would be smaller, less bright, less gentle without her in it.

Looking back, I can't fathom how I stayed so focused on all the tasks needing to be done. I had energy pouring into me that sustained me. I felt the presence of God with me all the time. I was in constant dialogue and prayer, asking for inner sustenance for Esther, Joe and I and everyone present with us. On the inside we were shattered, numb, empty but for Hannah, we kept our focus on preparing for the celebration of her short twenty-year-old life. We all had jobs to do, and we didn't want to let her down.

Hannah's funeral was planned for Christmas Eve. It was a miracle that it all came together in two short days.

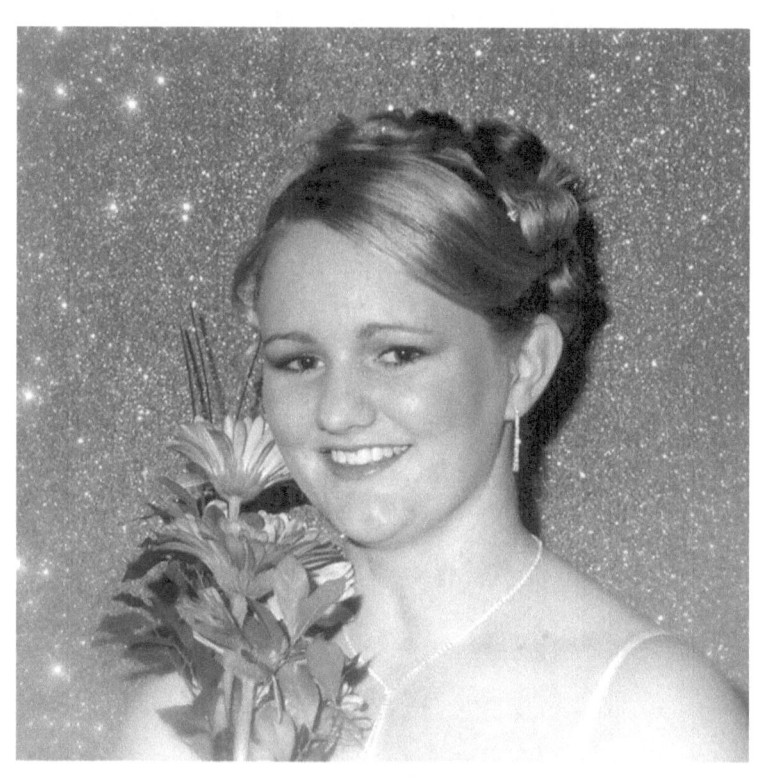

Hannah Rose at her St Paul's Debutante
Ball 2006 Kempsey NSW

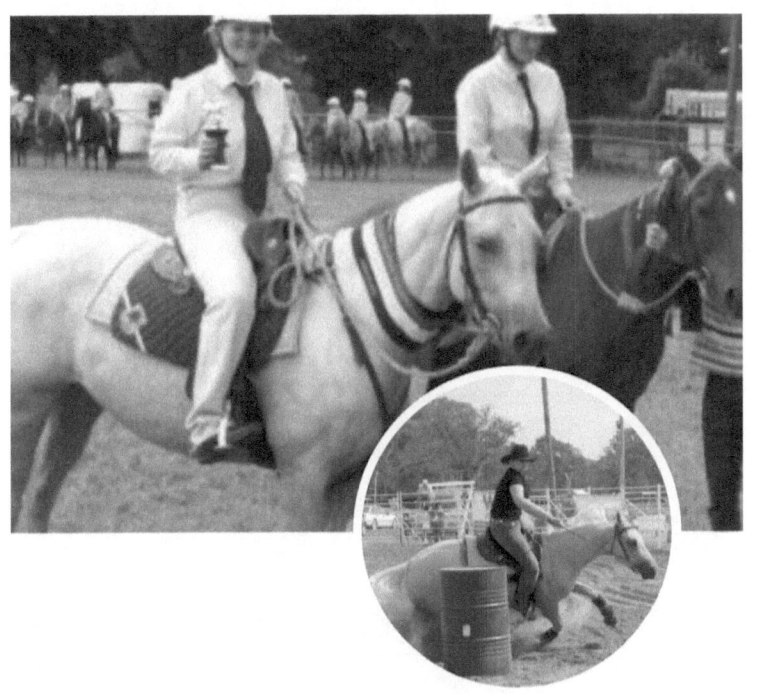

Top: Hannah, with Lena,
Zone 9 Campdraft Champion U21
Bottom: Chiltern Rodeo VIC 2008

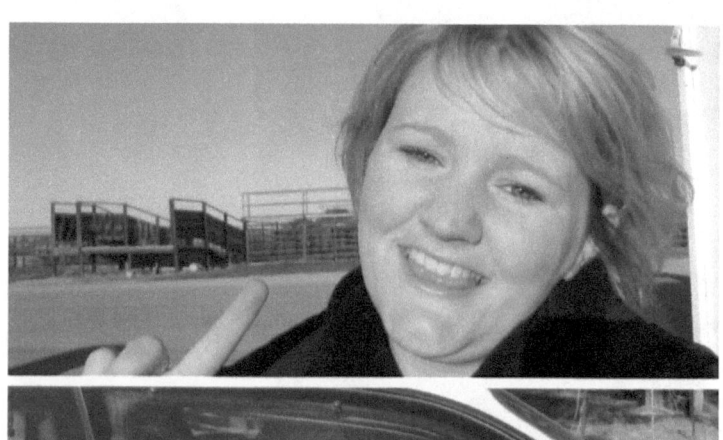
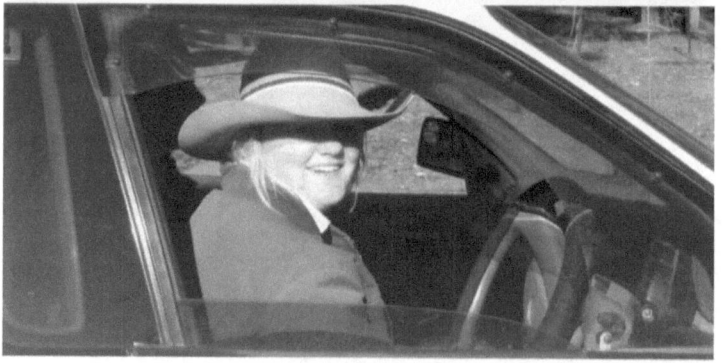

Hannah doing what she loved, travelling and her beloved Holden ute.

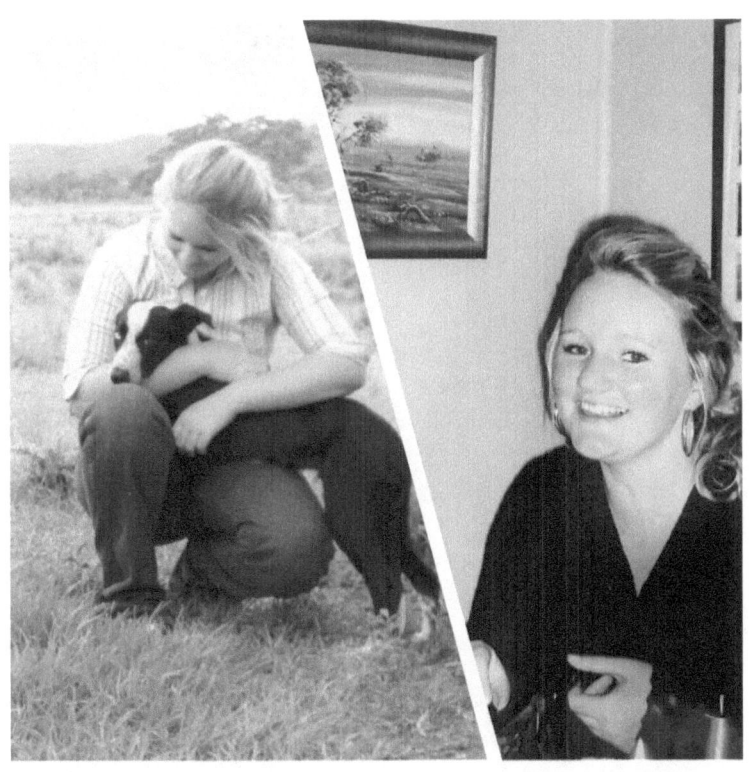

Hannah aged 19 with dog and 20th birthday 2008.

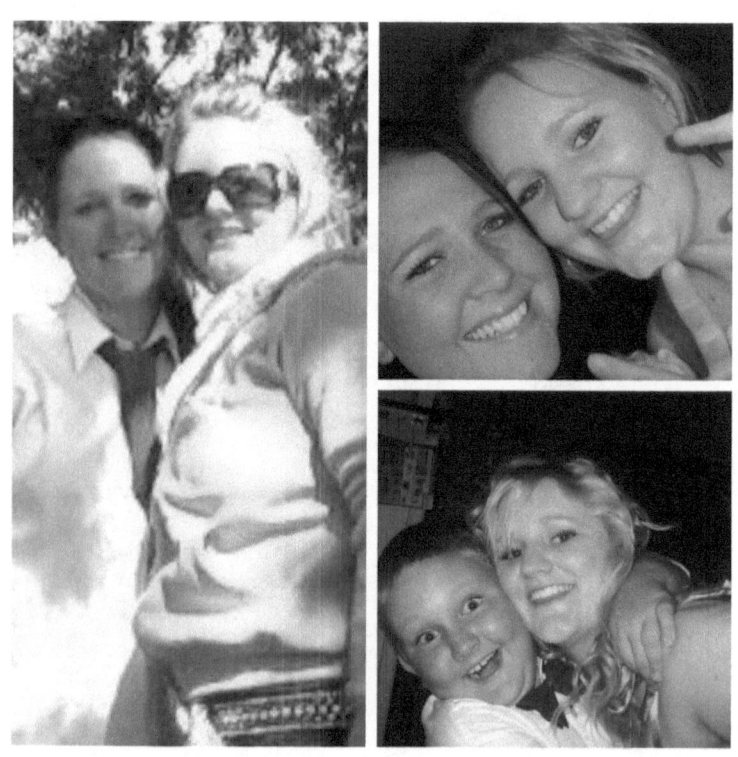

Esther and Hannah, Joe and Hannah.

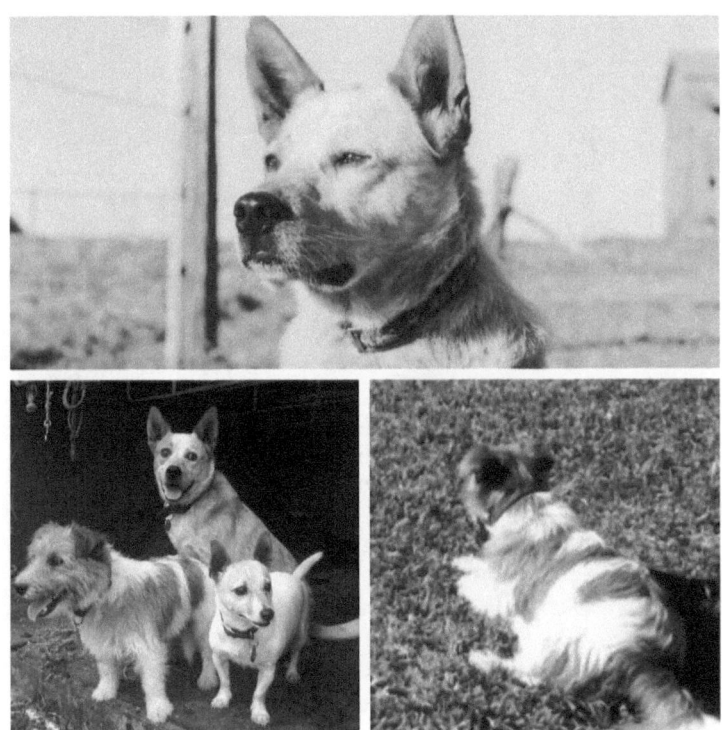

Dog Crew- Top: Bobby. Bottom left: Hamish, Bobby & Clancy. Bottom right: Hamish.

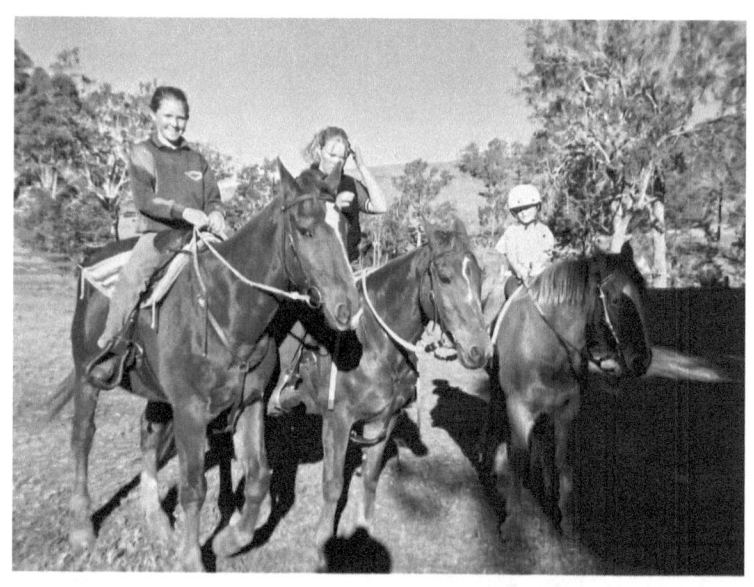

(L-R) Esther on Curly; Hannah on Bertie and Joe on Gruggie.

Chapter 14

Eulogy Flow

I had sat down the night before the funeral to write Hannah's eulogy. It didn't flow in the way I wanted. I prayed the words would come and went to sleep at midnight. At 4 am, I was woken up by one word echoing in my mind: Write.

Write I did. I had a computer beside the bed and I wrote like a whirlwind. The rhythm of the words and phrasing came out perfect. No edits. The words flowed gently out for an hour. My heart was on fire. Eulogies are important as the story of a beloved's life. I wanted Hannah's story to reflect her extraordinary short life, with some of her nuances and brilliance.

My first-born child made me a mother, made Lindsay and I parents. There was something profoundly grounding about that, and I wanted to honour that threshold to parenthood. Of all the things I've achieved in my life, being a mother is my richest. It came like a second skin. I loved every minute and never in all my years of parenting resented or wished it away. I've always had solid relationships with all three of my kids underpinned by respect.

When Christmas Eve came around, the funeral directors arrived at Kate's to place Hannah's body in her coffin and then in the hearse. That was no easy feat. When Hannah arrived from hospital to Kate's, she was on a narrow stretcher that was easily carried from the vehicle into Kate's lounge room, via the long hallway. This time with Hannah now in her coffin, it was another story. Kate had low bookshelves all the way along the passageway past the bedroom doors. The coffin didn't quite fit. It felt like a little Laurel and Hardy moment. All this effort and in the end, we couldn't get her coffin out of the house. We had a little panic to begin with and then got to work and had to do some quick rearranging of household items to make space and the men had to lift the coffin above the bookshelf to get it out.

Hannah was settled into the vehicle. It was a big black hearse with long windows the length of the coffin. The second funeral car was a black saloon sedan. We nicknamed it the Mafia Staff Car. My feelings were a mix of love, appreciation and foreboding about the day, however, at this moment we were buoyant that everything had fallen into place. We followed in the funeral car they provided for us. Joe was thrilled because there was a built-in esky in the back full of cold drinks and snacks!

It was incredible that we'd got things organised. The thought of Hannah going to a morgue for two or more weeks over Christmas and New Year holidays was unbearable. Plus, many of Hannah's closest friends and families were already in Melbourne as they'd come as soon as we knew it was end of life for Hannah. No hesitation. All of my family were around. It made good sense.

Darcy's mum and dad had travelled down from Queensland to support him. He truly thought Hannah was his life partner and they talked about their future together. This was a tough gig for any boyfriend.

I'd let those that couldn't travel to Melbourne for the funeral know that we'd have a memorial mass in Kempsey at All Saints Church when I returned.

The trip from West Melbourne to Saint Brigid's Catholic Church in Gisborne, where Father Michael would celebrate mass, took about fifty minutes. We arrived with more than a couple of hours to spare with plenty of time to decorate the front of the church and arrange photos. It had been meaningful for all who'd been at Kate's for two days to see and be with Hannah; we had an open coffin in the church. It felt inclusive of her being open to her own ceremony.

Several hundred people attended the funeral and Saint Brigid's was bursting at the seams. Out the front of the church, Hannah's mare Lena was tied up to the side of Mick's horse truck and her dogs, Hamish and Bobby, likewise.

A young person' funeral is different. The order of life is turned upside down when our kids die before us. Many of the young people wandered in and stood alongside Hannah, placing special things in the coffin.

I had dozens of people say the phrase to me, "You're living every parent's worst nightmare, Maura." I never knew how to respond to that and still don't.

Hannah's funeral was a mixture of joyous celebration and deep grief. They swirled together, inseparable emotions.

I remember many segments of the funeral. A powerful one was of the moment walking into the church. A moment I never thought I'd have to live. Walking into a church for my own daughter's funeral. Never, ever imagined having my child die before me.

I had moments where I said to myself, remember this. Tuck this away. I paused in the doorway and looked out at all the vehicles. So many utes, trucks, farm vehicles and cars.

This was Hannah's community travelling on incredibly short notice hundreds and for some, well over a thousand

Eulogy Flow

kilometres. This is the sign of a life well lived. A life that truly connected with others. My grief was she only had twenty years. That we, her family and community, wouldn't get to see the maturity of her life, except in our minds dreaming into that what may have been.

What made my heart sing as I walked in was Lena, Bobby and Hamish. All waiting patiently at Mick's truck. They knew what this day was. They knew their special human was no longer earthside and that Esther, Joe and I would be second-rate humans compared to Hannah for them.

The funeral mass was moving, with so many loving tributes. Father Michael felt like part of our family having said Mum's and now Hannah's funeral masses.

I'd met Father Michael in 1985 when I was only 23. The chain of events that led him to be standing in St Brigid's about to say a funeral mass for my dead daughter was too crazy to believe. When I was contract mustering and droving out the back of Hay, twenty-four years prior, I'd had a spiritual experience that bought my heart alive in a way I couldn't ignore. I was droving a small mob of 500 steers for Barry Hodgson, out west of Hay on my own. A local priest at St Fergal's in Hay, Father Alan Curry, used to go out into the remote areas and say Mass in pubs, shearing sheds, anywhere people gathered. He was 'God with skin on' to many.

ride4acure ORIGIN STORY

I was camped on the Hay Plains near Oxley; it was dead flat and barely a tree on the horizon. Lignum and saltbush grew in clumps across the plains with low box trees signifying dry creeks in the distance. To some the Hay plains can be empty, desolate. To me they made my heart happy, a great expanse of openness.

Fr Curry pulled up at my camp in his old car and wound the window down. I was just tying my horse Tom, a small brown stock horse to the side of the horse float.

"Put the billy on Maura, God told me you need to have a yarn with me!"

I was dumbfounded. Speechless. I was busting to talk to someone about what had happened to me on the inside, an unfolding inner journey, but there was absolutely no one in my working world I could do that with.

Here I was, an hour's drive from Hay on a remote dirt road, and a funny, down-to-earth priest just happens to call in. I did as he said and put the billy on to make tea. And then the lid came off my held-in feelings and words and I shared what had happened.

"Maura, one day this life won't be enough for you. Cattle, horses and dogs will no longer be your centre. God's got work for you in Hay. When you're ready come see me," Fr Curry said to me after I finished my story.

And as he sat back in his seat, an old 20-litre oil drum, he smiled at me with such light and sincerity that I almost believed him in that moment.'

"Father, that will never happen, this is my life. It's what I love," I replied.

He smiled even more and his eyes sparkled. He looked at me, right into my soul. It was the first time anyone in my life had looked at me like that. He saw me. Me. As I am. A cowgirl, a drover, living in solitude in the middle of nowhere. Happy with her life. However, he saw more for me, a much richer life that included more people.

It took less than twelve months for his prophecy to come true. I eventually went to see him and he gave me work in town with young people at the Hay War Memorial High School a couple of times a week and a job caring for the gardens of the Elders in Hay. I loved this new life. Rich and fulfilling in ways that surprised me.

Within six months of making the move into Hay, Fr Curry asked me to be the youth representative of the Forbes Broken Hill Diocese to attend the Youth Easter Retreat in Sydney at St Ignatius Loyola College at Riverview, Lane Cove.

It was a week-long retreat with young people under 25 coming from every diocese in Australia. It was a privilege. However, I suffered greatly from imposter syndrome. I was 'wet behind the ears', as my dad would say, and I felt completely under qualified to go. I was a rank beginner in the spirituality space, but alive with love, and my heart on fire and focused on living a more committed heart-centred life.

It was an incredibly rich experience, but one of the highlights was meeting a crew of Jesuit priests. One Irish priest, Fr Patrick O'Sullivan, was a good friend of my mum's and I'd met him when he visited Hay. He called me over to a table he was sitting at to introduce me to some other priests. There was a young bloke sitting there, barely thirty.

"Now Maura, what do you think of our hot, young soon-to-be priest, Fr Michael?" Father O'Sullivan said in his thick Irish brogue.

I literally spluttered out loud and I could feel my neck and face heat up and I knew I was going bright red.

"A waste Father, a waste," I said, saying out loud what I was thinking to myself, as I embarrassingly, walked away. I was shocked the words in my head came out of my mouth. I prayed the earth would open up and swallow me whole.

"I thought so Maura, I thought so," Father O'Sullivan said and gave me a big smile as I walked away.

Somehow Fr Michael's and my paths have crossed several times throughout my life. When Hannah died, he had recently returned from working overseas and was back in Melbourne.

Eulogy Flow

Here he was standing in St Brigid's with us yet again, about to celebrate yet another Luxford life, this one leaving earth too early for us.

Each of my nieces and nephews had a segment of the ceremony to manage and were all prepared. Each element went seamlessly. Our efforts in Hannah's funeral were acts of love for her and each other.

Incredibly I was present throughout the mass. I felt so grateful to read to each soul in the church in Hannah's eulogy. It felt like a gift for us all to share in that day.

When it came time to walk from the Church to the cemetery, about one kilometre. We all proceeded on foot with Hannah again in the hearse, followed by Fr Michael, Esther and Lindsay leading Lena and the dogs out front, and all of us trailing behind. We figured with a hearse and priest out front, we were less likely to get in strife for commandeering a road. We didn't seek permission from anyone, we just did it.

Drivers found diversions around several hundred people walking slowly in funeral possession, led by a glistening palomino mare, saddled for her last ride, wearing a massive garland of colourful roses toward the final resting place of her human.

The littlest kids had baskets of rose petals and they were scattering them along the road for us all to walk on; horses, humans and hounds. Rising above us was the sound of our voices, talking and laughing.

When we reached the cemetery, Hannah's place was the last row at the edge of bushland next to her cousin Max.

The year before Hannah's death, she and I were attending the funeral of a friend, Anne Holberton, in Bellbrook. Anne was a horsewoman, a farmer, and a highly regarded doctor in the bush. Anne had been one of my students in a mature women's Full Circle Horsemanship course I ran through Kempsey TAFE. Anne wanted to keep increasing her skill base and asked Hannah to continue on with her at her farm in Millbank using one of Anne's own horses.

Hannah took the job and gave Anne natural horsemanship lessons at her own property for over six months until she went to uni. Hannah would catch the school bus up to Bellbrook, give the lesson and stay overnight and Anne would get her to the bus stop the next morning. Sadly, Anne died tragically following a farm tractor accident not long after. Her funeral was in Bellbrook.

Hannah was only seventeen at the time and we were both standing in the Bellbrook cemetery after the burial.

"Mum, when I die, make sure I'm buried facing trees, looking out please, like Anne here," she said in all seriousness.

Eulogy Flow

"Don't be ridiculous, Hannah, like you're gonna die before me?" I said emphatically.

"Mum, I mean it," she said with an air of finality, giving me a side eye look, with a set on her face I hadn't seen. She was staunch in her stature at that moment.

I thought she was being maudlin because of Anne. I gave her a 'hmph' sound in response and looked out at the trees. How wrong I was.

I have a saying that guides me in life and I call it 'Metal Filings'. I imagine a powerful magnet underneath a flat surface that can be moved around, and on top of the surface, a random pile of metal filings. The magnet represents an intent and the metal filings are all the components needed to come together to make that intent come to life. The stronger the intent, the more metal filings are drawn to it.

The strong intention that Hannah's funeral would happen before Christmas and that all the resources needed would come together, was living proof of this principal. Evidence was us, a group of family and friends with Hannah and her horse and dogs, walking, as one, together, down the road toward the Gisborne cemetery.

When we arrived at the graveside, the reality of that deep, deep hole was confronting. Hannah's coffin was placed over the grave. A group of men including her dad Lindsay; her uncles Joe, Buster and Mick; her cousins and Darcy. The men, with incredible gentleness, held those green belts with tenderness and strength and lowered her ever so slowly down into the bosom of the earth as Father Michael's prayers poured forth to all of us and committed her to the earth. Her final resting place, her grave, near her cousin Max, was facing a large stand of gum trees, just as she'd asked me at Anne's funeral.

The baskets of rose petals and rose buds were offered by the little ones to all those gathered. Family and friends with this simple gesture offered a blessing carried on the wings of flowers and soil, into the grave.

Mick had arranged half a dozen shovels and by our own hands, we buried Hannah. In 2006 at Mum's funeral, after she had been committed to the earth with Dad, all nine of us, her children, were standing with others around her grave. Mick eyed the backhoe in the distance that would be used to fill in the grave. In that moment he said out loud, "Find a shovel. We'll bury our own."

On that day, with one shared shovel, that huge pile of soil disappeared into Mum and Dad's shared grave. It was a profound act of care.

This time at Hannah's burial, we were better prepared with six shovels and spades on hand already driven into the pile of soil. After the final blessings, the filling-in began. It was a physical act we all contributed to. It felt so satisfying as the hole slowly filled to know from beginning to end, we

Eulogy Flow

had honoured Hannah with our hearts and hands to see her laid to rest, looking out at her trees.

A thoughtful person had ducked down to the bottle shop and picked up a few cartons of icy cold beer and when the last shovel of dirt was complete, all of us stopped and stood simply staring at this pile of soil that now contained our Hannah. We slowly moved away and sat under trees in the shade and had a cold beer.

A peace settled over us all there, scattered about, some silent, some talking. All reflecting in our own way that one of our own was no longer walking earthside with us.

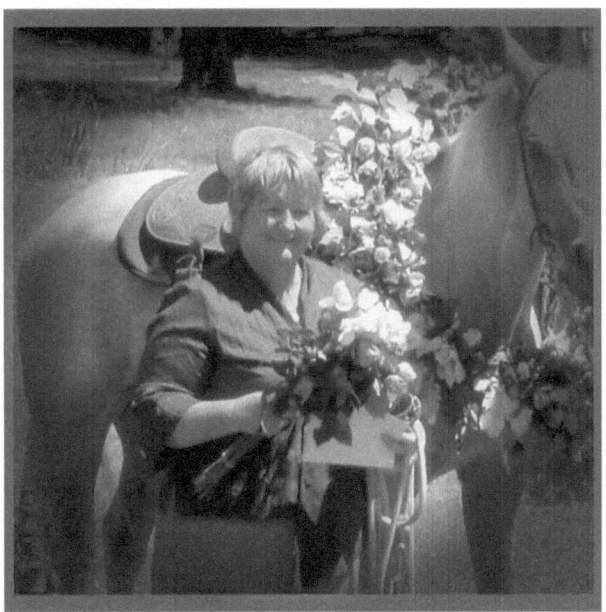

Maura and Lena, funeral procession with garland of roses. Gisborne Vic.

Chapter 15

The Wake

We gathered for the wake at the Gisborne Pub and the yarning continued. After an hour, I was ready for some quiet time. Trish, Joe and Jim were leaving, and I asked for a ride back to Kate's. There was a spare key hidden out the front and I could let myself in. Joe was with his cousins and Esther and he would come back to Kate's with them.

I remember sitting in the car in the back passenger seat, as we made our way along the Calder Highway back to the city, about a 50-minute drive. I looked out the window the whole time as I had rivers of tears flowing that I couldn't stop. I could hear the low hum of conversations about directions and best route to take, however it felt like it was happening somewhere else a long way away and there was a vast amount of space between me and the voices.

I felt all the air had gone out of me. I wanted to physically fall into the earth with Hannah. Not be on this side of it living without her. Yet I had Esther and Joe. My incredible other kids who I needed, and they needed me. I had to be here. That was final. Not negotiable.

After what seemed like an eternity we arrived at Kate's and I got out and thanked my family for the ride and watched them drive away.

I went to the front door and looked for the spare key. It's not there.

I've got no phone. No money. No Hannah. I sank to the verandah floor with my back against the door, curled up and cried my heart out.

It was Christmas Eve. I felt so alone. Bereft. Hannah was gone.

A while later, the woman from the terrace next door came out and asked me if I was okay.

"No, I've just buried my daughter. Kate's key isn't here, and I'm desperate for a cup of tea," I said sadly.

All this was said crying. This down-to-earth woman came into Kate's yard and put her arms around me. We silently

The Wake

hugged. She was crying too. After a while, in the gentlest voice, she invited me into her home and made me tea as I sat at her kitchen table.

Both of us sitting there with our hands wrapped around our mugs when she shared that her twenty-year-old son had died suddenly only a few months ago. I sat and looked at this soul of a woman before me. The relief and shared sadness that I felt in my heart was palpable across the table pouring toward me from someone who knew this. I didn't have to say a word. She knew in every cell of her being.

"I don't know how Maura you will get through this time, but you will," she said gently to me.

Someone eventually got home with a key and I went into Kate's place.

Kate's house quickly filled up with people. There were about twenty of us crammed into the lounge room, which had somehow had a complete transformation back to a living room, not a dying room.

Every surface had a human sitting on it, and many were on the floor. Before long, people started chatting about Christmas and what they were going to do the next day on Christmas Day.

My god, it was Christmas Eve. I hadn't thought about anything other than Hannah's funeral. I had nothing. I was completely empty.

Joe was sitting on the end of the couch with some of his cousins, who were excitedly talking about Christmas stuff. He looked lost. Kate realised that all the kids had Christmas things for the morning and Joe had nothing. Santa hadn't quite got his stuff together as Joe, like Esther, had been so immersed in Hannah's journey of leaving us and earth, that there had not been a thought of Christmas stockings or gifts for Christmas morning.

We realised we didn't care one bit about Christmas, only that it felt impossible to ever think about wanting to celebrate it again. Ever. Not without Hannah with us.

Joe had just turned ten the month before. He said many times, he didn't want anything. His ten-year-old heart was broken. Esther went and stayed with Lindsay that night, out west of Melbourne, out of town.

Joe and I were sharing a bed. Kate had offered us her double bed that night and we took ourselves off into the bedroom. Kate's family had gathered and were doing their best to have some kind of preparation for their own Christmas. I felt like I was in an alternate universe. I felt trapped now. Contained. Suffocating. I needed to escape, to get Joe and I, into the open away from everyone. Out of the city.

Before going to sleep, I called Lindsay and arranged that we would go to Charlton first thing in the morning, Christmas day, and pack up Hannah's things and sort her horses

The Wake

out. He agreed. Joe would go with Esther in Lindsay's ute and Lindsay and I would go to Charlton in Hannah's ute. Lindsay would go on back to Ivanhoe with Lena. Joe, Esther, and I would stay in a motel at Swan Hill for a few days and gather ourselves.

I couldn't stay in Melbourne for another day.

I was done.

With that arrangement in place, Joe and I went to bed, and both fell into a deep sleep. It was Christmas Eve. I had a ten-year-old boy and not a thought about Christmas, or how we would survive what lay ahead.

I remember waking up the next morning. I felt like I'd been run over by a B-double truck. My head was thick with fog, my heart heavy with grief. My arm asleep with pins and needles, and Joe snuggled into my belly. I didn't dare move. My bladder was chockers, and it was a long walk through the length of the house and garden to the outdoor loo. I managed to extricate myself from Joe's limbs and climb down from the bunk double bed without waking him. Kate had her work desk underneath her bed. I climbed down the ladder and snuck out of the room and crept quietly through the still sleeping house.

Barefoot, I walked down to the loo. On my way back to the house in this pre-dawn light, I looked up at the cityscape and glimpsed low-lying stars still visible. I was overcome with emotion and doubled over crying right there, under the grapevines. I begged God to help me. How was I to keep going?

"I can't do this, I can't!"

I'm sobbing to the early empty morning. What was going to happen to us? Then I had an image of Joe alone in the bed and I got myself together. I screwed my bare feet into the ground a little more and took a deep breath and moved myself slowly back inside.

I made mugs of Milo and tea and headed back to Joe. He was sitting up cross-legged on the bed holding a very poor excuse for a Christmas stocking in his hand. He looked so sad, but then he broke out into a grin and said,

"Santa's hit a new povo level this year, Mum," he smiled. "He's resorted to a servo Christmas stocking."

He held up a plastic net Christmas stocking, full of throw away stuff and cheap lollies. Somehow, it made it all a little more heartbreaking. Joe laid it on the bed unopened and we drank our hot drinks.

I shared with Joe the plan to simply pack and get on the road and for him and Esther to do a road trip in Lindsay's ute. He was totally lined up with that plan and hitting the road as soon as we could pack.

The Wake

Esther and Joe were to go on to Swan Hill. Lindsay and I would meet them there at sunset, all going to plan. I had booked a motel for a few nights for us to regroup. They were keen about having a swimming pool at the motel to funk around in and to finally be on our own.

We were ready to leave family and Melbourne forever, for us, the last place we saw Hannah alive.

Having tasks lists to do was a relief. I kept focused on the next thing.

When Lindsay and I arrived at Charlton, I set about packing up Hannah's things and Lindsay managed her saddlery and horses. It took us the good part of the day and we would just make it to Swan Hill before sunset.

Hannah had a fluffy pink cushion and matching blanket with a shag pile look. I rolled it into a bundle and kept that out, as it smelt like her. I sat it on the console of the ute between Lindsay and I as we drove away from Charlton. Lindsay looked at it when he got in to go. He didn't say a word. He knew.

We drove in silence for about twenty minutes. I was driving and towing the float with Lena on board and the dogs. I was looking straight ahead when a cop car pulled past me and put lights on for me to pull over. I was doing twenty kilometres over the speed limit in an 80km zone.

ride4acure ORIGIN STORY

The cops in the Charlton area are deadly on speed and notoriously hard-arsed about fining people.

"Do you realise you were speeding? Are you the registered owner of this vehicle?" The cop said as he came to my window.

"No officer, I didn't, and no, I'm not", I stuttered.

I promptly burst into tears. Head forward on the steering wheel, full on sobbing.

"Maura and I buried our daughter yesterday. We've just packed all her things up here at Charlton. We're trying to get to Swan Hill before dark." Lindsay gently said to the officer.

I slowly lifted my head from the wheel and wiped away my tears and blew my nose. The officer genuinely looked at us both with such care, "Drive safely. Pay attention to speed. The next cop may not be so generous."

He paused then said, "I'm so sorry for you both." He said the words that I have since heard hundreds of times: "You're living every parent's worst nightmare", as he tenderly patted the roof of the ute.

We know.

On cue, at sunset, we drove into Swan Hill to the motel. We'd already dropped Lena at the showgrounds in a stable

The Wake

for the night. She was fed and tucked up. I'd talked to the motel owners about having Hamish and Bobby in the vehicle for the nights and given the circumstances, they made an allowance for us.

When I drove the ute into the motel carpark, it was such a relief to see Esther and Joe playing in the pool mucking around like little kids playing 'Marco Polo'.

We organised takeaway food and sat outside in the BBQ area and ate together. Esther and Lindsay shared a room and Joe and I, the other one. The next day, Esther's friend from Port Macquarie would come to pick her up and take her back to Port with Bobby. Lindsay was taking Lena back to Ivanhoe, and Joe and I heading back to Kempsey.

It came time for us all to part. Lindsay and Lena to Ivanhoe, Esther back to Port Macquarie, Joe and I to Ellenborough. Joe and I were in Hannah's silver Ford BA ute. We had decided to stop and fish along the way. We found some great spots on the Murray River to fish and swim. We'd bought a handline, some tackle and frozen prawns. Joe fished, or as he'd say, "fed the fish". I slept. Deeply.

I was so exhausted. I had to stop frequently to have ten-minute power naps. I hadn't slept for so long during the whole time Hannah was in hospital. My body, mind, and soul was exhausted. We were driving along and I looked sideways at Joe. He had rivers of tears flowing down his little boy cheeks. I simply reached out and laid my hand on his arm. No words.

"Mum no one is ever gonna love me like Hannah did," he gently said through his tears.

"That's true Joe, that's true."

I didn't sugar coat his truth. It is what it felt like in that moment and was true for ten-year-old Joe.

Hannah was his big sister. His guiding star. Our guiding star. She lit up our lives and was gone now from our visible worlds.

I had arranged with Steve and Patricia, Esther's and Joe's Godparents, for us to stay at Ellenborough for January 2009 in their retreat accommodation. It faced the stunning Ellenborough River. We needed a place to land and regather. Ellenborough was perfect.

Esther threw herself back into work and was riding track work at both Port Macquarie and Kempsey. She was living with a female jockey in Kempsey in a two-bedroom flat and was supplementing her track work by giving riding lessons to adults in between track and training.

Esther was giving horsemanship lessons to a student on a farm out on Nelson's Wharf Road at Aldavilla, west of Kempsey. While we were staying at Steve and Patricia's, Esther had a phone call with the owner of a property she was giving lessons on. The owners were moving to a property at South West Rocks.

The Wake

"If you ever want to rent your farm out," Esther casually said to her client, "Mum, Joe and I would like to rent it from you."

I had nowhere to live. Before Hannah had died, I'd temporarily moved back to the farm, living separately. It wasn't ideal. I'd done that so I could continue delivering my Full Circle Horsemanship courses at the farm. It worked for Joe, as it meant not having to go between two parents. However, now with Hannah's death, this was not workable for me.

Chapter 16

Gap Month - Ellenborough River

We were homeless, rudderless. We had collected Joe's dog Clancy from the farm. Clancy was the only pup of Hannah and Esther's first little dog Michelle, a Jack Russell, chihuahua, fox terrier cross and he was with us at Ellenborough. Joe loved Clancy; we all did. He was like a second skin to Joe, never far away, they were inseparable.

My good friend Janine Taranto came to visit us at Ellenborough and we all went down to the river for a swim with the dogs. Clancy was swimming and playing with Joe. The next second Clancy disappeared. We couldn't see him, but we could hear him. His bark was coming from underground on the opposite bank of the river. Janine and I swam across and tried to work out what was going on.

"Don't let Clancy die Mum!" Joe said getting more upset. He kept repeating this over and over as Janine and I were trying to feel down holes in the riverbank for him, ripping away at tree roots to get our arms further down holes hoping to get our hands on some part of Clancy's little body.

Eventually, with Joe now in a full-blown panic attack, sobbing out of control and Patricia trying to comfort him, Patricia had the foresight to suggest they go to the house to get dog treats for when Clancy was rescued. Janine and I frantically continued our dog rescue. Janine's long skinny arm finally found the tiny foot of Clancy.

"I've got his foot Mauz!" Janine said.

"Get hold of his bloody leg and don't let it go. Pull as hard as you can even if you break his leg, pull him out. He can't frigging die in here Janine, get him out," I said under my breath.

In my mind's eye, I saw him clawing at the dirt in the tunnel trying to hunt whatever creature he'd followed down the tunnel. As hard as Janine was pulling his leg, he was clawing forward to get the animal and fighting to get out of her grip. Eventually, just as Patricia and Joe were returning with treats.

Gap Month - Ellenborough River

"He's coming out!" Janine yelled excitedly.

Joe jumped in the river and swam the ten metres across to the opposite bank to Janine and me. Under the momentum of Janine's vice like grip, a mud-covered Clancy came out of the hole backwards and leapt into Joe's arms.

"You're alive Clancy, you're alive." Joe sobbed over and over.

Janine, Patricia and I looked on. We knew what a miracle this was and together uttered a prayer of thanks that Clancy was okay.

That was enough drama for all of us, and we retreated back up to the cabins for afternoon tea and naps.

Chapter 17

Returning Home

While at Ellenborough, we'd started planning Hannah's Kempsey Memorial Mass. We selected Valentine's Day 2009 for the Mass. I had made arrangements for Father Adrian Stephens from Christ Church Saint Laurence in Sydney, to concelebrate the mass with my good friend Father Chris Chaplain MSC.

I worked with the kids' old school, Saint Pauls and their friends. I put notices in the Macleay Argus and gave people plenty of time to plan to travel to make it.

Hannah, Esther, and Joe's friends all worked together with me to create a reflective ceremony that honoured Hannah and the short time she'd spent on earth.

Willawarrin Pony Club did a guard of honour at the front of the church. A group of school friends had gone out to Temagog, Toorooka and Bellbrook to gather river stones from Hannah's favourite swimming spots on the Macleay River to use in the ceremony for the altar procession. In the communion preparation, all the young people in the church had either a river stone or rose in their hands and carried it to the front of the church and laid it at the altar. This long snake-like procession of young people contributing to saying farewell to one of their own was moving for all to witness.

Dixie Chicks' *Wide Open Spaces* blared over the sound system along with other country favourites of Hannah's. The DVD of images looped on the church walls.

To begin the memorial, a group of Dunghutti Elders, all women, grandmothers, led us in a Welcome to Country, and a water blessing. They shared words that recognised the relationship we had and the care they held in their hearts for us. I felt truly blessed, finally at home. The words, the singing, the blessings; I felt Hannah's spirit being called home to this country. This country that had nurtured, loved and held her through her childhood.

The women walked the aisles of the church using branches of red flowering callistemons dipped in bowls of Macleay River water and with branches held high over their heads flicked water droplets out across the whole congregation aisle by aisle. One of the Dunghutti Uncles performed a smoking ceremony. The richness of these symbols was

Returning Home

profound, coupled with the heartfelt Memorial Mass that followed with Fathers Adrian and Chris. Everything about this felt perfect and good.

The mass was a profound simple ceremony that recognised the continuation of Hannah's soul beyond her earthly journey. The prayers, the rituals all for thousands of years one way or another have bought comfort to people in times of deep sorrow and joy. For generations my own family had leant into these rituals and beliefs. For me they have been like navigational tools helping me stay on track through the toughest and most joyous times of my life.

It was a moving, reflective celebration of Hannah's life in her hometown of Kempsey and beloved Macleay Valley. The church was packed to the rafters and spilling onto the streets. The Macleay Argus, the local paper, wrote a story about Hannah's funeral which featured on the front page.

The final week before the memorial, Joe and I had been living with Esther and her friend, in their two-bedroom flat on Crescent Head Road. Joe had his swag on the floor in Esther's bedroom. I slept in with Esther. Most nights, Joe ended up in with us both. We were waiting for the Nelson's Wharf Road home to be vacated at the end of February, and we had a lease to move in after the memorial. That was perfect for us all. We could have our horses and dogs there with us.

The home was on the Macleay River, surrounded by lush farmland. It was perfect. It had a garden and of course the first thing I did was set about getting some veggies in the ground. Joe got into gardening too and growing food with me. Almost daily, Joe would ask me, can we ride our horses again yet? I couldn't. I literally broke open, going near my horses. Lena came with us when we moved to this farm. I could care for them on the ground, brushing, rugging, feeding but I simply could not ride. I couldn't fathom never riding with Hannah again.

One day, when Joe had asked for the hundredth time about riding, I said, "Well, I can't ride horses yet, but what else can we ride Joe?" "Mountain bikes Mum," Joe said. "Mountain bikes." "Good idea, let's do it." I said.

That afternoon we went into town in my BA Ford ute and bought what I thought was two flash Giant mountain bikes and a bike rack and got it fitted to the back of the ute before we took the bikes home.

We started with short rides down the dirt road, but after a few days were riding further until after a week or so we're going into Greenhill to the shop about eight kms each way. I said to Joe how about we get fit enough to ride into St Joey's and that he could ride his bike to school. That was a plan. That was fourteen kilometres each way. Joe jumped at it. Within a few weeks of riding every day and clocking up the kilometres, Joe and I easily rode into Saint Joseph's. I would meet him there in the afternoon after school, and we'd ride home together.

Returning Home

Joe was in Year 5 and had Mr Z as his teacher. Mr Z had taught both Hannah and Esther and had sung and played guitar at Hannah's memorial. He was one of my kids' favourite teachers. On Joe's first day at his class, I'd walked Joe up to his class. Mr Z saw us outside the classroom and he came out and he simply wrapped Joe and I up in his big strong arms and hugged us at the same time. He said to Joe with his hand on Joe's shoulder,

"I've got you Mate." And with that, Joe walked into the classroom. Mr Z looked at me, hugged me again, and walked back into the class. No words. We both knew.

A few things happened at this time. I started to think about my promise to Hannah to get fit again and I realised that while I was riding the push bike, I didn't think about anything. If I felt my grief while riding, I'd switch my focus to my pedals and focus on pedalling harder, stronger, fuller. Pedalling to the next white post only and not thinking past that.

All I was focused on was riding. Turning the pedals, staying alive and being with Joe. I was fairly unfit at this stage, so feeling my body getting stronger every day was a good thing. When I wasn't with Joe or Esther, I was crying. I didn't believe it was possible for so much water to exist in my system. I had rivers of tears pouring out of my eyes a lot of the time when alone.

ride4acure ORIGIN STORY

I couldn't turn this off. Early in March 2009 I rode my push bike into town after riding with Joe to his school. This had become a daily habit for us now. I had decided to sign up at a women's gym to fulfil my promise to Hannah to get fit again. I rocked up at the gym and signed up. I was weighed, measured and walked through a fitness plan and mapped out my goals. It was pretty simple. Get fit again.

The machines were set up in a circle on the gym floor and I moved robot-like around the circle, methodically going through the motions, thinking about Hannah all the time while I pushed and grunted through some of the moves. I cried endlessly in the gym. I didn't care if people looked at me. Most everyone in town knew of me and it was well known my daughter had died. Kempsey town itself is a small rural town of only ten thousand people and almost thirty thousand in the entire Macleay Valley.

I went to the gym every second day. I started to look forward to going, as it was one more predictable thing in my life. The last year had given me my fill of unpredictable living. I'd had a gutful. I wanted a known, measured, planned life from now on.

After about a month of being at the gym, I was reading the posters on the noticeboard while working out. One was advertising a women's financial planning session through the Macleay Valley Business Womens Network. I was in dire straits financially and was on a Centrelink payment. I had taken leave without pay from TAFE as I couldn't go back to teaching and didn't know when I could.

Returning Home

My then boss at Kempsey TAFE had invited me to his home for coffee to talk about returning to work and a welfare check, I think. He was an excellent gardener, and I was absorbed in his stunning garden. We were standing on his verandah, shoulder to shoulder, both looking at the spectacular views. In the foreground, his stunning semi-formal gardens full of perennial flowering plants; toward the river a well-organised vegetable garden with a backdrop of the mightly Macleay River, framed by the Great Dividing Range in the distance.

As we stood, he quietly asked, "Are you closer to being ready to return to teaching Maura?"

I turned my head to look directly at him, deep into his eyes.

"Mate, a team of bullocks couldn't drag me into a classroom."

I said emphatically, "I don't know if I can go back. I've lost my mojo."

And with that, I cried.

My currency in the classroom indoors and out had been my connection to my students. I had a big heart for the complexity they overcome to get themselves to study again as I worked mostly with youth at risk. After Hannah's death it was hard for me to be around people who struggled with valuing the precious gift their life was. I experienced my own dark night of the soul as challenging thoughts swirled in my consciousness.

Throughout the year of Hannah living with melanoma, not once did she say, "Why me?" Not once.

I made up for it in the time after her death. In my pain, grief and heartbreak I fought and raged with my God. At moments, I was furious with anger that she was gone forever physically from my world.

Hannah who had so much to live for. Dreams, hopes for her career, friends, family, horses, travel, relationships, marriage, babies, holidays. All gone. It stopped with her death. I knew so many people who didn't care about the privilege of having breath in their bodies. Didn't value time on earth. I couldn't at this time in a teaching capacity be present authentically. That was the currency of my credentials as a teacher. I genuinely had loved what I did.

I'd lost my mojo, and I didn't know at that point if I'd find it again.

Chapter 18

A Man is Not a Financial Plan

I looked at that noticeboard in the gym and saw the tagline on the poster which said, 'A man is not a financial plan!' I actually laughed out loud at that. I thought of how in my life, my financial security was tangled up with the success or failure of marriages. I was shocked when I heard a loud sound, and realised it was my own laughter. Here I was two months after burying my daughter, laughing out loud in a public place. I figured I needed to go to that forum. Anything that could get me to laugh at this moment was worthy of my time.

ride4acure ORIGIN STORY

It was a good investment of a few hours. That workshop began building my financial literacy and helped me put foundations into the next chapter of my life. It got me connected to a great bunch of local women from the Macleay Valley Women in Business, many of whom I remain friends with.

My background in social science and community services landed me in teaching roles at TAFE in Humanities, Community Services and Women's Studies. Interestingly, when I first returned to study in 1990, the first course I did while I was still droving was New Opportunities for Women or NOW. I did that through Adelaide TAFE via correspondence and loved every minute of it.

I'd got booted out of one of the worst high schools in NSW in the late 1970's as a teenager in Moree and hadn't done any study since. I loved study and once I started with Adelaide TAFE, I didn't stop. I ended up studying women's studies, literature and social science at uni and loved every minute of it. It was a full circle moment when I started teaching for TAFE NSW in 2001 at Kempsey Campus. I was well credentialled and quickly employed to teach the equivalent of that very first course I'd studied myself a decade earlier as a drover in Western NSW.

What I learnt about myself during those times was how profoundly deep my resilience is. My capacity to remake, rebuild my life through the toughest times wasn't just a thought, I was living proof. I had a deep trust that things work out for me even in my darkest hours.

A Man is Not a Financial Plan

This was the bedrock I kept coming back to as I navigated the time directly after Hannah's death.

Timing is everything. My confidence, empathy and love helped my kids make transitions that were tough. I knew in my bones if I was aligned with my choices. If I'm okay, my kids would be okay. There was no room for guilt or shame. My kid's wellbeing was closely tied to my own. I needed to get grounded and focused. They looked to me as an anchor and I needed to be present.

I felt my grief and sadness deeply, however I kept connected to the earth and everything around me.

"Don't be sad for me Mum, I'm gonna be ok", Hannah's heartfelt words that she repeated to me daily during those last weeks echoed around my brain all the time.

Many times, I wanted the earth to crack open and swallow me. To stop spinning and let me get off. I hated being in the world without Hannah in those early months of grieving and was full of disbelief that on the outer people were privileged to be going about their days like nothing had changed. Whereas for us, our whole axis had shifted off centre in our world without Hannah.

At this point in my life, my sister Veronica was the only other person I knew well that had lost a child. She was a rock to my aching heart during this time, a safe place to lean into and be supported.

ride4acure ORIGIN STORY

A couple of months after Hannah's death, I was lying in bed, my arm hanging down the side, crying quietly with my eyes closed. The doona pulled up to my chin with rivers of tears flowing over my face into my ears. I didn't care. There were so many tears I'd given up wiping them away. They simply flowed uncontrollably when I was alone.

However, I wasn't alone.

"Mum, I don't know what I'd do if anything ever happened to you," I heard Joe clear his throat and say in his ten-year-old voice.

I was dumbstruck at the clarity of his words and the power. Like lasers they went into my heart and pierced me. I shuffled over in my bed and threw the doona back to invite him in.

"I'm not going anywhere Joe, I'm here with you buddy, like you and Ezzie; sometimes I'm just so sad about Han and I can't stop the tears."

No more words were spoken. We simply laid in bed holding each other and dozed off.

In another life as a counsellor and transpersonal therapist, I knew the impact on kids of sibling deaths. Statistically, the rates of self-harm, suicide, addiction and drug abuse are diabolical after the death of a sibling. I was aware of this and it was a key driver for me to be as present as possible and involved in both their lives to the best of my capacity while navigating and honouring my own journey through grief.

Fortunately for me, I have a solid friendship circle of souls that know me and welcomed me just as I was.

I was a member of the Australian Transpersonal and Emotional Release Therapists Association and did a retreat at Douglas Park around Easter 2009, only a few months after Hannah's death. I spent most of my time reflecting and crying, but one thing I did was a vision quest led by my good friend Fr Chris Chaplin. It was an experience. Pre-dawn walking into the bush, granite escarpment territory, with only water for an extended period from 4am for a day. The night before the vision quest, I'd had a profound dream where Hannah had visited me and she was wearing a pair of green 'Wizard of Oz', Dorothy shoes, all sequins and magical. I was planting seeds in a garden and she was sitting beside me with her glittering shoes on, sharing with me that she was now everywhere… I felt her so powerfully and knew this to be true. She was alive in me and those that held her love in their hearts.

Finding a place where I could be, without expectation, was a catalyst for me to be as present as possible. The vision quest gave me a deep experience to be with myself and the power of the gift of the dream, feeling Hannah everywhere and, in my heart, energetically alive. This brought me deep joy. However, I could equally move quickly from that feeling into grief that was still overwhelming at times most days.

ride4acure ORIGIN STORY

Those first months were heart breaking. Most days bled into each other. The milestones for me were getting the bikes, signing up for the gym, getting my body back in the pool, and swimming. These three physical activities helped me stay focused in the present moment. To be as present as I possibly could for Esther and Joe.

On my solo bike rides, large white birds similar to the ones in the hospital window on the day Hannah died, started appearing. On fence posts, flying in front of me for periods of time, like a string pulling me forward. They would fly in a direct line ten metres in front of my bike at helmet level. I felt they were calling me forward to keep going. Some days I'd want to stop the ride but the birds were flying in front of me so I kept going. I couldn't leave them. They were elegant, graceful birds. Always alone. Which is how I felt, rattling around inside myself. Alone with my grief.

My friends were loving and kind but grief is, I learnt, predominantly a solitary journey.

My sister Veronica made the long drive of 1500 kms from her home to mine to come stay with us for a week. I was so profoundly grateful for this generosity. Not long after that, I was surprised when my childhood best friend from 1968 when we were six-year-old girls at St Mary's in Bairnsdale, Mary-Lou Capes, with her older sister Sue, drove from Stratford in Victoria all the way to my place at Kempsey.

A Man is Not a Financial Plan

"Guess where I am?" Mary Lou said, as I nearly died hearing her voice.

"I have no idea," I said, "Surprise me."

"Kempsey," Mary-Lou said.

I shrieked. I didn't believe her as she was welded to East Gippsland. I couldn't fathom that she'd driven all the way to see me with Sue. I was beside myself with joy. I gave her directions out to our little farm and before long we were sitting at the kitchen table drinking tea.

The world is changed by those who show up. At that time having people show up to simply be with me made a huge difference and healed a little of the gaping cavern that was my broken heart. I am forever grateful to everyone who stood alongside me and my kids and loved us through that tough time.

I wrote endlessly in my journals, spilling words on the page to lessen the heart burden. I drew, gardened, cooked. I kept doing normal things and when not, I was on my bike riding kilometres a day.

I couldn't see a white bird and not think of Hannah and how she left Earth. In my garden at Nelson's Wharf Road on the Macleay River, I had many moments of feeling Hannah's presence. Mostly with small birds and butterflies making themselves known to me in a personal way, a new way. I felt the gentleness of her spirit close to me and it gave me a profound sense of love in my heart.

It reminded me of a reading from my mum's funeral in 2006 from a poem called, Togetherness.

Death is nothing at all.
I have only slipped away into the next room.
Whatever we were to each other, we still are.
Call me by my old familiar name.
Speak to me in the same easy way you always have.
Laugh as we always laughed at the little jokes we enjoyed together.
Play, smile, think of me, pray for me.
Life means all that it ever meant.
It is the same as it always was.
There is absolute unbroken continuity.
Why should I be out of your mind because I am out of your sight?
I am but waiting for you, for an interval somewhere very near, just around the corner.
All is well.
Nothing is past.
Nothing has been lost.
One brief moment and all will be as it was before – only better.
We will be one, together forever.

Canon Henry Scott-Holland excerpt from 'Death is Nothing at All' (1910).

Henry Scott-Holland

Chapter 19

Beyond Grief

I was grateful Mum and Dad were dead.

The agony of losing another grandchild would have been an unbearable burden for them both. What I knew from Hannah's dying is they were definitely present with her, with me. In Hannah's hospital room, there was a sense that the room was full of energy. I could sense my parents and my maternal Grandma, Winnie Pollard, my good mate Ginger Burden, my nephew Maxie and others, waiting, supporting.

I had shared this with Father Michael Smith, one day remarking that the room was crowded. I explained I could *feel* them all in the room on the right side of Hannah's bed.

Lined up shoulder to shoulder. Sentient guardians to carry her home. He understood.

"They're all here." Hannah murmured to me repeatedly, confirming for me the unseen visitors in her room as she moved in and out of consciousness.

Hannah had nerves removed from her neck and arm with the last surgery that gave her a Mona Lisa smile that didn't quite reach her whole mouth. And her one arm couldn't reach above shoulder height. During her last days, she would smile a full smile on her semi paralysed mouth, and her long arm would reach out for an invisible hand, as if someone was helping her. Clearly for Hannah, someone was present and she was seeking support from them. Joyfully, she was illuminated each time she did this. She wasn't aware of me or anyone else. I knew something other worldly was happening for her and I was witness to this incredible moment. I simply attended to her needs as best I could and was present.

"Do you know how much I love you, Mum?" and "I'm going to be ok Mum, it's all going to be okay, " Hannah repeatedly said to me.

When she said that, she would reach up and gently stroke my cheek and smile deeply. I had soaked it all up. My heart breaking knowing I wouldn't get that nanosecond again. I replayed those moments hundreds of times as I rode alone.

Beyond Grief

Veronica, my younger sister, gave me sage advice about those last days to make every second count and to not waste a moment. She learnt this the hard way when her son Max died suddenly in a traffic accident in 1999. Veronica and her other children, Sam and Liz, didn't have time to say goodbye. It brings me some comfort to know that both Max and Hannah are buried in Gisborne cemetery next to each other. Cousins together, resting in peace.

As I rode my bike, I often tuned into standing in Hannah's hospital room knowing I'd not get a nanosecond of time back again. I didn't sleep for the last week of Hannah's life. I reflected on how I micronapped standing doing Reiki or sitting on her bed resting my hands in hers. I had felt myself energetically resting, even as I cared for her. I had taken emotional snapshots of my time with her and stored every frame in my heart. I wanted to remember everything about her. Her smell, the softness and gentleness of her touch. The wispy flow of her blonde curly hair. The sound of her voice. Her divine eyes, blue pools of curiosity and wonder. The translucency of her skin. I wanted to remember every little detail. And I do. My senses are full of her all these years later. Still alive in me.

I replayed those moments a million times as I rode one white post at a time on my bike, or swimming laps in the Kempsey Pool, or working out at the gym. In the replays, I was enthralled with how little I knew about what happened with dying.

ride4acure ORIGIN STORY

As a spiritual woman, with a lifetime of transpersonal experiences, that affirmed for me, the reality of my soul and the souls of others who I have connected with after their death. I have never doubted the reality of the continuation of Hannah's soul's journey after leaving earth.

Chapter 20

Talking About Our Dead

Stories fell out of our mouths. We talked about Hannah all the time within our family and we listened to each other, we laughed together and cried together. We were never tired of talking. Deep down while we mentioned her name, filled our house with visual reminders, she was alive with us. Her fluffy pink blanket and pillow that had sat in the front of her ute while we drove from Charlton back to NSW the day after Hannah's funeral, to this day sit on our couch at home and are cuddled, held or patted daily. It was one small way to remember our dead. To honour Hannah and acknowledge the place she holds in our family.

ride4acure ORIGIN STORY

Since the day she left us, I've burned candles in memory of her, had a small prayer table set up at home with other family and friends who left an imprint in my heart alongside her now too. Daily I remember the dead who, through their life, helped me live a deeper, richer more meaningful life. I pay my respects to them. Always. I remember them.

Something deeply organic happened in these early days. People with their own stories to tell found their way to me, often sharing their stories of loss for the first time.

One of the hardest to hear was mothers who lost teenage kids while their husbands and other kids didn't want to talk about them. It was like they were erased from their lives. Visual reminders cleared away so as not to bring up memories.

Everyone finds their own way after death. There is no right way.

Once I started doing radio and print interviews, people reached out and connected, many for the first time. Harrowing stories just like Hannah's. Stories of disruption, detours, delays and death.

A local family contacted me as their only son had died from melanoma not long before Hannah. I went to their home, and we sat at their kitchen table and over a cup of tea, shared stories and heartache. We cried together at the waste of our young one's lives that would never be lived and the empty place as parents that we don't get to see our children's lives unfold.

Talking About Our Dead

Some parents I met who had children that died, struggled to speak about their loss, so I simply sat with them. In the same way the woman next door to Kate's home in West Melbourne came to me and sat with me in solidarity as a parent who had skin in the game of death, at some visceral level, this brings comfort to know we're not alone in that often dark, endless void.

My son Joe when only ten years old, six months after Hannah died, told me a story about his school day when I'd picked him up after school. We were parked sitting in my Ford ute out the front of his school.

I asked him if anything weird happened at school that day. He shared that one of his less enlightened teachers asked him if anyone in the class burned candles at home or had an altar.

Joe's hand shot into the air like a rocket and he shared proudly the story of Hannah's altar. He shared that we'd set an altar space up on our kitchen bench. He described how it got rays of the morning sun. With photos of Hannah, flowers, feathers, special rocks Joe had chosen, some crystals. Meaningful symbols of love and curiosity. Often a toy or crystal would be placed there by Joe as "Han would like that Mum," he'd say. Always when we were home, a candle burned, to remind us of her light that lived on beyond earth. He enthusiastically shared all these details with his teacher and class.

ride4acure ORIGIN STORY

When the teacher asked Joe, "How long ago did Hannah die?"

Joe said, "Six months."

Surprisingly the teacher said, "Don't you think it's time to stop burning candles Joe?"

He didn't miss a beat and said with confidence, "Well Miss, Jesus died two thousand years ago and we still burn candles for him."

Joe was looking at me when he shared this with a sad smile on his face. I asked how he felt when she said that.

He wisely said, "I didn't feel angry because I knew she'd never lost anyone she loved more than herself Mum."

I knew my boy was gonna be okay.

He was working this grieving out in his own wise way.

Chapter 21

Lighthouse Moment

With every stretch, every step, every turn of the pedal, I loved how my body was beginning to feel. In a few short months of movement, to find space from the pain of grief, my body transformed from fatigued to fit and fabulous.

At the start I'd felt full of aches and pains. Everything hurt; my bones, muscles and heart. Over time, I felt more and more connected to Hannah and that fulfilment of getting fit. The fact that she died and didn't have that opportunity to continue to live in her human body made it more poignant for me that I celebrated living in mine and what a privilege to be in a body, to be alive and breathing.

ride4acure ORIGIN STORY

My fitness became my focus. I was riding my bike, going to stretch classes. Swimming a kilometre a few times each week, and for fun, aquarobics once a week with the elderly. I loved this and had heaps of fun. I would go to the gym and work out and then come straight across the road to the pool and swim. My day was focused simply on fitness.

The privilege of being in a body and feeling alive never left me. After living through the reality of my beloved daughter taking her last breath and closing her eyes forever, it fired me up to appreciate being alive. I felt that truly in my body. While I was swimming, riding, stretching and at the gym, I felt free and connected to Hannah.

"Oh, I saw you riding out near Clybucca," people would say to me as I was popping up everywhere in the villages of South West Rocks, Crescent Head, Bellbrook or Willawarrin.

I felt like Forrest Gump when he ran across America. I got on that bike and I just didn't get off. Fitness took me to a whole other place and level of presence.

While I was turning the pedals and moving my body, I wasn't drowning in grief. Physical movement gave me space on the inside and around my heavy heart.

Fitness became my medicine.

Esther was pre-training racehorses over at Port Macquarie and Joe would go with her and help on weekends to swim

Lighthouse Moment

horses. We had teed up that I would ride my bike to Port Macquarie and meet up with them after Esther finished work. It was a 140 kilometre round trip ride to Lighthouse Beach from home. I thought nothing of it. The longer the better.

The life-changing day that burnt into my mind and heart started normally. I left home on my bike before dawn and landed over at Lighthouse a couple of hours after sunrise. It was a three-hour ride for me each way. I rode up some steep hills to Lighthouse beach. I loved it. I was so fit I could just ride up anything. My lung capacity was mind blowing. I celebrated every win. I loved that there wasn't a hill I couldn't ride up. I had to use what I called 'Granny Gear' where my feet were spinning like crazy for an incremental forward movement of the bike but move it did. I love that capacity in me that transformed my body from fat and fatigued to develop a high level of fitness in a few short months.

The day that I rode to Lighthouse Beach was pivotal in this whole journey. At the lookout I got off my bike and leaned it against a fence. I was looking out to sea and was mesmerised by the waves crashing against the rocks. The sunlight left an incredible golden light shimmering on the water where birds were swooping and diving hunting for fish.

A soft, cool breeze was cooling my sweat. I stood transfixed, looking out to sea, thinking about Hannah. Thinking about the journey I was on as a mum and the support that I was giving to both Esther and Joe to help them stay in their skins while they navigated their own grief journey.

I could feel my heart getting bigger and bigger till it felt like my chest was going to burst. I thought for a minute I'd overdone the ride and was having a heart attack. Then I started softly sobbing. Overwhelmed, missing my girl so much, I thought in that moment I was going to die too. I couldn't bear the feeling in my heart. What had started as gentle tears turned into torrents rolling down my cheeks. I started crying out loud, snot crying, choking tears.

Then I heard, an audible male voice say, "Maura ride for a cure. Ride your bike to Peter Mac in Melbourne. Ride for a cure."

I was pulled back into the present moment, looking for the source of the voice. There was no one near me.

"Maura ride for a cure," I heard this distinctly. I was sobbing, crying, laughing all at once. I realised without a doubt, I could and I would.

I was shocked. I looked about because it felt like someone was beside me. There was no one except the tourists about five metres away, moving further away from the crazy bike woman.

"Mum, when we get through this thing you and I are going to do something to raise money to help find a cure," came Hannah's voice again with energy.

I looked out to sea and up to the clouds, putting my arms out and whooped a "Yes" to the Universe. I was so full of this

Lighthouse Moment

vision that embodied every cell of me. I could feel Hannah urging me. I could feel my spirit saying yes to the call to ride4acure. I knew in that moment I could do it.

"I don't understand this but I feel in my bones the rightness of it. I can do this. Yes, I will do this," I said to God, the universe, my higher power right then.

There was no room for doubt. Something bigger was at work through me.

I felt a circle of support around me that provided the fuel for me to bring this vision to life to ride to Melbourne, to raise money to find a cure, and to visit kids in schools. I knew I could do this. I felt myself come back into the present moment and looked around me and I realised that there were people about, and because I'd been making a bit of a racket, they were looking at me strangely. They had moved further away to put some distance between themselves and me, the loopy woman on the push bike. I felt energy come down through my head and into my spine, arms, legs and feet into the ground, receiving a charge of energy in every cell of my being.

Then I went totally quiet. All the strong energy faded away, and I felt like a huge pool of quiet, deep, cool water, full of peace and calm. The boundaries of my body expanded, and I felt limitless, floating, soft, and open. I felt Hannah with me, beside me and in me. Though she wasn't physical anymore, I felt her energy just as powerfully.

ride4acure ORIGIN STORY

My fuel was to remember the words she shared with me to: not be sad, to get fit again, do something to raise money to find a cure, and to tell all her friends. These simple phrases became my reason to be.

I had a lucid memory of Hannah in Sydney back at the start standing in the doorway to the surgeon's rooms facing each other. We were leaving and he told Hannah she was the luckiest girl alive as he'd just given her the 'all clear'. There were no cancer cells outside the surgical area.

"Hannah, tell all your friends to look after their skin, he said with his hands on her shoulders looking into her eyes.

"Yeah, I will, I will," she said convincingly. Those simple words stuck with me. Took root deep in my mind because over and over they came back to me, particularly after Hannah died and this day at Lighthouse Beach. It was like a bell going off in my brain. I could not stop this reverberating energy of the words, "Tell all your friends to look after their skin."

I could see all the other 'Hannahs' out there in rural and remote areas that didn't have someone to encourage them to look after their skin to help them understand why, and how important that was. Who's going to tell them and I realised in that moment it was me. I could do that for Hannah. I knew how to connect with kids; I knew how to work with the education system, especially in rural and remote areas. I knew without a doubt, it was the right thing for me to

Lighthouse Moment

do. I could do this. I had already ridden more kilometres simply getting fit than was the total distance from Kempsey to Peter Mac in Melbourne.

When I met up with Joe and Esther for breakfast that day, I shared with them all that had happened at Lighthouse and they one hundred percent backed me and would help me to bring it to life.

I don't remember the ride back to Kempsey. I barely remember the lung-busting ride up Mount Cooperabung. I rode home in record time to get on my computer and create a plan.

I sat at my kitchen table and thought about what I could share that would stick with kids and get them interested in their skin. I would create a multi-media presentation that was a mix of three things; storytelling around simple science, personalising it through Hannah's story and a call to action to kids and communities everywhere I would go to be part of finding a cure. It would be a community effort.

On a big piece of butcher's paper. I did two things. In a couple of hours, I mapped out what I could share in 45 minutes with a group of school students about melanoma and skin cancer prevention. I asked myself the important question, 'What would they need to know?' I had in my mind if Hannah had an opportunity at her school to have someone visit and speak about skin cancer and melanoma prevention, what would have made a difference for her?

That guided me as I researched simple science around melanoma prevention. I checked every single thing with the melanoma experts and put together a multimedia presentation.

A middle-aged, generously sized mum from the bush who, until recently, was well known for having her bum in a saddle on a horse. Now here I was planning to complete a bike trek from Kempsey to Melbourne. A journey of over 1600 kilometres as I went into many communities off the highways, including Canberra. Everyone I spoke to came on board and believed in me to make this happen. Waves of support flooded in from that moment forward.

The more I spoke about it, the more resources flowed. From that Lighthouse moment, I never doubted it would be done.

Within a few days, I went into the Kempsey bike shop. The two blokes who owned it had done a fair bit of long-distance riding. It was where I'd bought our bikes.

"Boys, I'm going to ride my bike to Melbourne. I'm riding for a cure for melanoma in memory of Hannah," I said and told them about my intentions to complete a bike trek.

"Let us know if there's anything we can do to help," they said in unison.

They looked at me and confirmed what I'd known that I had already ridden more than the distance to Melbourne.

Lighthouse Moment

And in fact, they said that when I got on the road it would be easier; that I was at the peak of my fitness and strong in every part of my body. There was no doubt in their mind that I could do it. And no doubt in my mind either.

Everyone I spoke to supported me. It was phenomenal. An extraordinary moment in time where I was free from doubt and that assuredness was mirrored back to me in my family and all I spoke to. If anyone thought I was completely crazy they never told me.

Ride4acure was supported by the Peter Mac Foundation to fundraise for the Hannah Rose Melanoma Research Fund.

I didn't know at this point what to call the multimedia presentation, however, about a month later I was at the Kempsey NSW Cancer Council Relay for Life community event. Joe and I were walking through the night in memory of Hannah and as well we had a ride4acure stall selling merchandise and raffle tickets. We had our ride4acure T shirts and Akubra hats on. I had a pull-up banner beside the ute that had ride4acure featured on it and a few words about the Hannah Rose Melanoma Research Fund at Peter Mac fundraising to find a cure for melanoma.

A little kid come up, standing there, not saying anything for a while. He was about eight or nine and he tipped his head to the side like a working dog trying to make sense of a command, looking at this weird word 'melanoma' on the banner.

ride4acure ORIGIN STORY

"Mela, mela, mela-what?" he said.

In that moment, I had chills down my spine and I knew that was what I needed to call the multimedia presentation. Mela-what? That was it. I knew exactly how the boy felt not to understand and to be bamboozled by a strange word. I felt that sitting in Doctor Carmel's clinic back at the start with Hannah and when I started to learn about melanoma. I had felt exactly like that little eight-year-old kid.

The name had found me. Ride4acure was the trek name, Mela-What? was the multimedia presentation name and the Hannah Rose Melanoma Research Fund auspiced by the Peter Mac Foundation. Everything was falling into place.

The job I settled into doing was the logistics. If I was to ride a bike to Melbourne, what resources would I need? I used another piece of butcher's paper and mapped that out extensively. When I saw the enormity and reality of this big audacious goal, one part of my brain for a second screamed, *how could you possibly do all this?* The support, the logistics, the resources, sponsorship, and to keep the massive training schedule up to stay fit. It was huge, and it was just Joe, Esther and me.

In that moment, looking at the huge mind map of the logistics on the table in front of me, I had the overwhelming energy that came to me at Lighthouse, as I stared at that mind map. My body was filling with it. I was infused with a vibrancy that felt incredible, and I knew I wasn't alone.

Lighthouse Moment

"Help me with this one. Please bring what's needed". I was filled with calm. This pattern repeated many times throughout that first trek preparation. I would have moments where I felt overwhelm and would come back to my centre, remembering I'm not alone. Feeling Hannah beside me every step of the way, every turn of the pedal, spurring me on to ride4acure.

I simply felt a deep and profound reassurance that all would be okay. I had trusted everything would work out. I asked for support, asked for invitations to speak about the trek, and kept fundraising and getting known. From that moment on, I had a steely knowing in my bones that the logistics and resources would work out. My job was to maintain a laser-like focus on where I wanted all this to land. And I knew it would come and that my job wasn't to make it happen, it was simply to identify the detail to the best of my ability and trust that what I needed would come.

Metal filings. Trust in the vision of ride4acure. It would come. I did the logistics and resource list. I daily did whatever it took to stay in my energy, to keep focused on the goal and Hannah's wishes and to allow the resources to make this trek a success flow toward me. My job was to stay centred, connected to the why, to be strong and, keep training.

This was the point where I had to split my attention. I had to maintain the rigorous and demanding training schedule, work on the logistics and the sponsorship. It was massive.

ride4acure ORIGIN STORY

I broke the logistics down into segments and did the same with the invitation and itinerary for the schools.

I had connections in the communities I was traveling to with strong connections with local Rotary clubs. They got me connected to many other clubs along the way that invited me to speak and facilitated fundraisers for ride4acure. I planned to ride down the main highways to Melbourne via Sydney and then to Canberra and then back out to the Hume Highway via Yass. I went where I was invited. I said yes to everyone. I gave presentations at schools, Rotary Clubs, Lions Clubs, sporting clubs and gyms. Media invitations started to roll in as word circulated by word of mouth of the ride4acure bike trek from Kempsey to Melbourne.

When I accepted the call to ride4acure, I said out loud that I needed the right people to be put in my path. I would take massive action on training, talking with people, asking for help however I needed to find my tribe for this to become reality.

Calling in the resources needed to do the trek was a whole other mind-blowing experience. A life lesson in trust and openness. I believed with my whole self that what I needed would come.

I had five months to plan, gather the resources and fundraise. I'd set a target of raising $45 000 for the trek and to share the Mela-what? story with as many people as possible that would motivate them to look after the skin they're in.

Lighthouse Moment

The clarion-call was received at a place called Lighthouse Beach, a symbol of safety and a light in the dark. I received the message loud and clear with the call to action to create an entity called ride4acure.

As a woman first and foremost I leant into my intuition with my mind open and fuelled by grit. Every cell knew this was what I was meant to do at this time. This was the beginning of an epic journey that went far beyond trekking. I could not foresee then that my Lighthouse moment was an invitation that would ultimately bring me home.

Home was being as fully alive as possible while honouring those I love in life both on earth and off.

Home was honouring Hannah's two hopes to tell all her friends to look after their skin and to raise money to find a cure.

Home was sharing Hannah's story with all the other Hannahs out there, in rural and remote areas, in simple, memorable ways that may help them be curious about their skin health and the skin of those they love and motivate them to take preventative steps.

Home was feeling threads of love wherever I am that sustain me.

Home was knowing in my bones that death is a doorway and love never dies.

Afterword

My work with ride4acure encouraged people across the nation to be curious about the skin they're in. What science has shown us is prevention and early detection are our best tools to take care of our skin. They can prevent a significant amount of melanoma and skin cancer. Given that exposure to damage in the first eighteen years of life lays down the majority of what will happen on and in our skin for the rest of our life, early education is critical.

Encourage your friends to be curious about their skin.

If you're in a clinic at a skin check, never let a doctor say, 'lets watch it." It's your skin. Your life. If you're worried enough about a spot to get yourself to a doctor, ask them to cut it out and request it gets sent to pathology and tested.

All the experts agree that early detection is key to survival. To this day I question the first time Hannah asked a doctor about the new spot under her ear, had they had cut it out and sent to pathology for testing, what difference could that have made to her survival? It was six months later when I saw it and booked her into to Doctor Carmel who went full ninja on it. I loved her for doing this for us. For taking rapid action. For recognising the signs.

I have such love and deep respect for Dr Carmel who, sadly, died suddenly a few years ago. In her memory, I planted a hedge of eight white rose bushes that I can see from my writing desk. Carmel was and still is in my heart and mind, a legend of both a woman and rural doctor.

I did ask our amazing melanoma specialist that very question. He sagely counselled me to 'not torture myself'. All these years on I still wonder. I mull that over now and again. The fact Hannah asked doctors twice, told me her intuition knew it needed looking at. To think a ten-minute procedure to remove it may've saved her life. We will never know.

Before Hannah's diagnosis, I had so few people in my life that had lived through major health disruptions. After Hannah's death, they came out of the woodwork. Daily people and their stories found their way to me.

A layer had been peeled back to show me this web going on below the surface in every community. Families dealing with life-changing moments, doing what they can to keep things going all the while playing a balancing act of

Afterword

caring for loved ones, working and contributing to their community. They're the true unsung heroes and often fly under the radar. Reach out to those doing it tough. Let them know you care.

We are more powerful, stronger and resilient than we know. It is through the pressure of life experiences that I've connected to my grit, my inner strength to persist in the face of profound adversity, while keeping my heart open and living as a woman with compassion for others, the land and environment I'm on and immersed in.

Show the people you care about how much you love them and let them know.

You never know what's around the corner.

Acknowledgements

With respect and gratitude, I acknowledge that I write this book on the unceded lands of the Dunghutti nation and pay my respects to the traditional custodians of this land where I have raised my family, loved, worked, grieved and lived for over three decades. I acknowledge the love and respect my family and I have been welcomed with here.

I acknowledge my family the Luxford clan, and all of my siblings, their partners and the two dozen plus nieces and nephews. Family is my 'reason why' in life.

I acknowledge my three kids, Hannah, Esther and Joe. They are the lights of my life.

I am grateful to both my husbands, Lindsay Matthews and David Collett. Because of you I have the blessings and joys of my life, my children.

ride4acure ORIGIN STORY

Deep gratitude for my parents, Marie and Kevin Luxford, for the lessons learnt over many years droving livestock and living in remote areas and most importantly, how to value family. That life experience developed droving and living in the bush gave me a deep sense of capacity within. I knew how to get things done, to trust where life meets me.

Limitless gratitude for Jeannie and Adrian who opened their hearts and home to us for months at a time in Sydney. They lovingly held us as we navigated the unknown, providing safe harbour in an unfamiliar city. They gave us practical love with warm comfy beds and hearty food to keep us strong, and lovingly held our hearts and minds during tough times, giving us a home and a place of peace and renewal.

I am deeply grateful for the extended community stretched across the nation that have reached out to me and encouraged me over the years with ride4acure.

To the many hundreds of people who asked me to write the story of ride4acure, thanks for your encouragement and I'm delivering on that promise with book two due out in summertime 2024.

To the incredible medical staff in every hospital and clinic across our nation, I honour you. You never know the impact you may have on patients and their families. I'm forever grateful for the love and care shown to Hannah and my family during the toughest of years. Thank you.

Acknowledgements

Dr Carmel Shanahan (dec.) you were (are) a legend to me. You took action, gave strong and clear directions and loved us through the toughest of times.

I have such deep respect for writing mentors along the track including stand out, Stephanie Dale, of the 'The Write Road'. Steph has been supporting women in the bush in rural and remote areas to write on country. I had the great privilege to attend a women's writing retreat at Paka Station, Lake Mungo in 2022 that fanned my writer's spark. We've had touch points over the last decade that have left an imprint in me.

Heartfelt gratitude to Natasa and Stuart Denman and the team at Ultimate World Publishing. Your support and mentoring made the dream of publishing possible.

I acknowledge the power of great teachers. One of whom planted a seed in me, Val Clark at Narrabri Tech in 1978 who told me I could write and to not stop.

Thanks to you Val, I've kept at it ever since.

I acknowledge grief as a teacher. A relentless, powerful, ruthless teacher. I have gone places both within and in my outer life because grief knocked powerfully on my door. A different grief to the death of my parents and other family members and friends. A grief that entered my very bones. From the ashes of that grief, I have found depths of life unimaginable to my old self.

ride4acure ORIGIN STORY

I acknowledge the push-pull, love hate relationship I've had with the Catholic Church over my life and the deep love and respect that resides in my heart for the spirituality I live that is tangled up in it. I have had the good grace to meet the living heart within those who are sons and daughters of the Church and am grateful.

The testament of the holy men and women I've journeyed with has given me such a deep taste of love and the heart of God in action. They are my *God with skin on*. I acknowledge Fathers Alan Curry (dec.), Chris Chaplin MSC, Fr Adrian Stephens, Michael Smith (SJ), Patrick O'Sullivan (SJ), Steve Nolan (dec.). The Presentation Sisters from Hay and Wagga in the 1980s who taught me what real prayer is in the thick of life and my heart sister Patricia Nolan, who every day demonstrates the simplicity of love in action.

A final word about writing this book. I have had a lifelong dream to write and publish. I acknowledge my gritty drive and sense of humour. In April 2023 I was having a self-satisfied moment when outside in the garden laying on the soft grass looking up at the sky through the leaves on my mulberry tree. I was reflecting on how fulfilled in life I was in that moment. I was feeling a sense of wellbeing that I had achieved the key things I'd wanted in life and if I were to die tomorrow, I'd die happy.

Out of nowhere I heard a voice with a strong judgmental tone saying, *Nah Maura, you didn't write the fucking book, did ya?*

Acknowledgements

Oh my God, I didn't! I laughed out loud recalling the many times I was asked, "when are you writing the ride4acure story Maura?" and my response was, "I will down the track." End of April 2023 was my 'down the track' moment. I made a commitment then and there, to write a first draft by the end of August and publish. To keep myself on track I made a consequence that would be a stretch for me if I didn't keep my word. I've been growing my hair for a couple of years and my favourite hairdresser Emma, has been helping me with crafting my Suzi Q layered style. I decided that if I didn't have a first draft by end of August, I would shave my hair off. I went to my hairdresser the next day and said exactly what I've written above and that if I didn't write the book, she'd have to shave my head. And in her busy salon in front of customers and looking me right in the eyes, she said, "I'm not shaving your hair off Maura, you're gonna write the fucking book!"

Thanks Em, you're a champ, here it is.

About The Author

Maura grew up in a large family of nine kids. Her playground, the travelling stock routes of Victoria and New South Wales, droving livestock with her parents Marie and Kevin Luxford. Much of her primary education was by correspondence in the 60s and 70s with her mum as her teacher. In the late 70s, Maura got kicked out of one of the worst high schools in the state and finished Year 10 droving out the back of Bourke with her dad and 1400 head of cattle. Despite that, she graduated from university twenty years later with a degree in social sciences. Since then, she's had a long career in community development and education.

Horses and livestock held significance throughout her life including seven years running Full Circle Horsemanship where hundreds of students came through a self-leadership and communications program using horses. The classroom was their farm at the foot of Mount Sebastopol in what is now the Willi Willi National Park. This thousand-plus acre outdoor classroom was the ideal environment for young and old students to reset and reconnect to life and their community.

ride4acure ORIGIN STORY

Maura calls the Macleay Valley home and has spent over thirty years living on Dunghutti Country and is now on fertile acres on Euroka Creek just out of town.

When not at her day-job, she's planting habitat trees, growing food and flowers, sipping tea, watching birds and wildlife in her garden or off on an adventure on her motorbike.

For over twenty years, Maura has worked in vocational education and remains passionate about its transformational power.

For her social and community work she was voted:

- Social Entrepreneur of the Year in 2012
- Woman of the Macleay Award in 2012
- Oxley Woman of the Year in 2013
- She was inducted into the International Long Riders Guild for her solo packhorse trek with her three incredible horses Meg, Billy and Wrangler in 2010, where she rode over 1800 kms from Kempsey in New South Wales to Melbourne Victoria, 'the long way.'

Her greatest achievement in life is being Mum to Hannah, Esther and Joe.

Humans she's proud of.

Book 2 Due Out Summer 2024

Book 2 Due Out Summer 2024

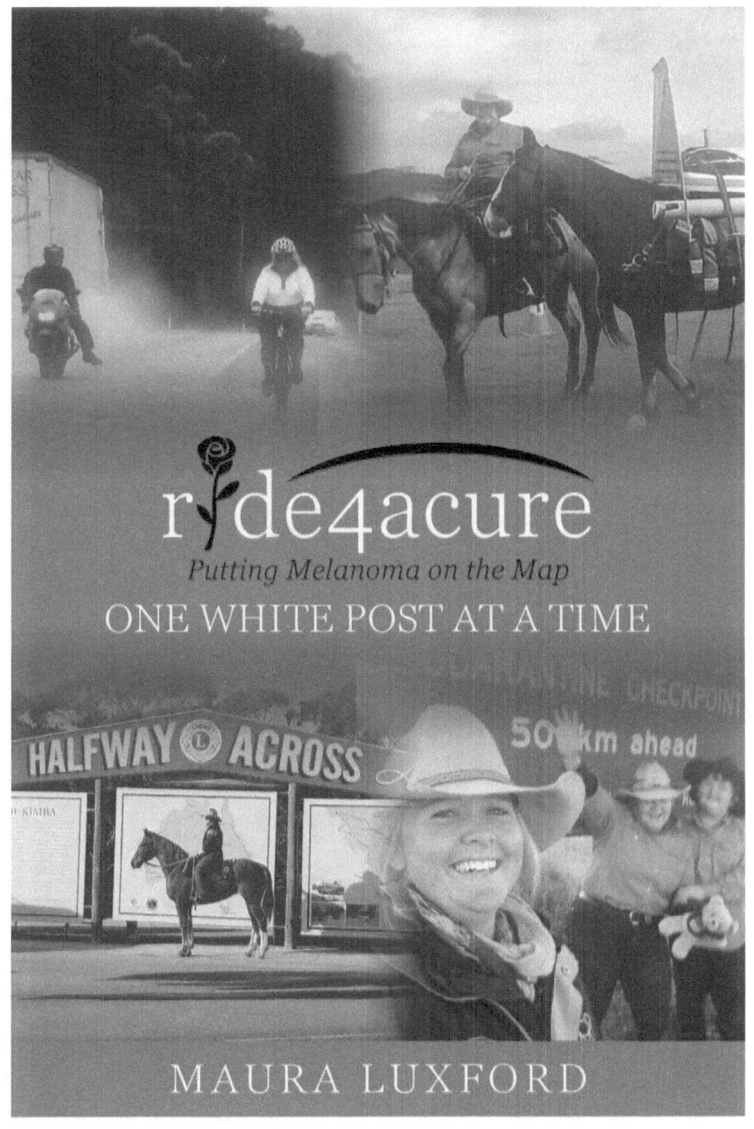

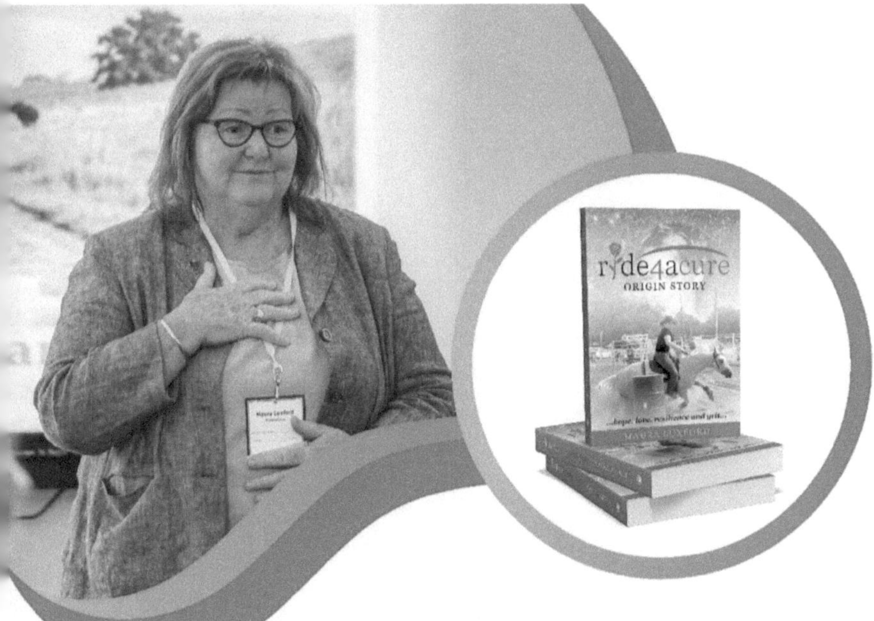

Speaker Bio

MAURA LUXFORD

Five years, five states, one hundred and fifty schools and raising $150,000 advocating for health literacy about one of the most prevalent cancers in young Australians, was the life work of ex-drover, educator, mother of three and social entrepreneur Maura Luxford.

Fired by the death of her eldest daughter Hannah, and bringing to life Hannah's two dreams of 'to tell all her friends to look after their skin', and to 'do something to raise money for research into adolescent melanoma to find a cure', changed the course of Maura Luxford's life.

Creating a social enterprise called ride4acure, Maura scaled the breadth of our nation. Traversing Australia on horses and a push bike to some of Australia's most rural and remote areas to speak to young people in their communities.

Over time, navigating her way through the tangled path of grief has reshaped Maura and enables her to speak with confidence and authenticity in the space of loss, death and grief.

- ✓ Loss, grief and dying
- ✓ Melanoma and skin cancer prevention advocacy
- ✓ Living with grit

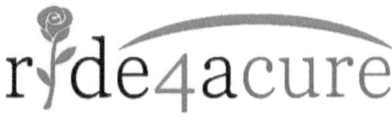

 www.mauraluxford.com.au   *maura.luxford@gmail.com*

Book Club - Questions for Readers

1. What was your favourite part of the book?
2. What was your least favourite part of the book?
3. Did you find the author's story compelling? If so, why?
4. What do you think motivated the author to share her story?
5. Which part stuck with you the most?
6. How did the book compare to other memoirs you've read?
7. How did the memoir make you reflect on your own life?
8. Would you want to read another book by this author?
9. If you could ask the author anything, what would it be?
10. How did this book impact you? Do you think you'll remember it in a few months or years?
11. Are there any lingering questions from the book?
12. What did you learn from hearing this author's story?

Notes

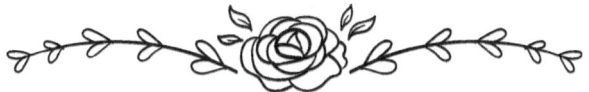

_____

_____

_____

_____

_____

_____

_____

_____

_____

ride4acure ORIGIN STORY

Notes

ride4acure ORIGIN STORY

Notes

www.ingramcontent.com/pod-product-compliance
Lightning Source LLC
Chambersburg PA
CBHW030257100526
44590CB00012B/432